THE POLIVAGAL THEORY & DAILY VAGUS NERVE EXERCISES

2 IN 1: LEARN HOW TO REFURBISH YOUR BRAIN AND YOUR BODY THROUGH DAILY EXERCISES TO REDUCE INFLAMMATION, ANXIETY AND CHRONIC ILLNESS

REINER HARTMANN

REINER HARTMANN

CONTENTS

BONUS CHAPTERS
The Gut-Brain Connection & Healing Your Child's Vagus Nerve

WHAT THIS BOOK ISN'T AND WHO MIGHT WANT TO PASS

While we're bursting with excitement about the potential benefits of diving deep into this bundle, we also believe in transparency. Let's lay out what you shouldn't expect from this journey and who might feel this isn't the right fit.

What Not to Expect from This Book:

- **Instant Miracles**: While the techniques and insights shared can be life-changing, they require time, consistency, and practice. There's no 'magic button' for instant results.
- **Medical Advise**: This book offers wellness insights based on research and experiences, but it isn't a substitute for professional medical advice. Always consult a healthcare provider for health concerns.
- **Technical Jargon Overload**: We've tried to keep things light and easily digestible. If you're looking for a heavily scientific treatise on the Vagus Nerve and Polyvagal Theory, this might not be it.
- **One-size-fits-all**: Every individual is unique. While we offer a range of techniques and insights, not every strategy might resonate or work for everyone.

Why This Book Might Not Be For You:

- **Looking for Quick Fixes**: If you're seeking instant solutions without committing time or effort, this book may disappoint. Real change is a marathon, not a sprint.
- **Medical Professionals**: Those with advanced knowledge in the field might find the information too basic or general. We aimed to make the topic accessible to everyone.
- **Skeptic of Holistic Approaches**: This book leans into holistic wellness and the interconnectedness of body and mind. If you're strictly in favor of traditional medicine, some sections might not resonate.
- **Not Open to Exploration**: We encourage readers to try various techniques and be open to new experiences. If you're not in the mood for exploration or trying out new exercises, this might not be your cup of tea.

THE VAGUS VOYAGE!

Hello, dear explorer! Ready to navigate the intricate twists and turns of your body's very own superhighway? Let's unpack what this bundle offers, but don't worry— I've ditched the jargon and kept the fun.

- **Meet the Vagus Nerve**: This isn't just some fancy name to impress at parties—it's your body's very own "command center." We'll break down its roles, why it's got celeb status in the world of nerves, and how it plays a sneaky hand in those Monday blues or Sunday euphoria.
- **Polyvagal Playground**: Hold onto your hat because next, we'll unravel the mysteries of the Polyvagal Theory. Imagine having a cheat sheet to your emotions—knowing when they're about to swing, dip, or soar. That's what the Polyvagal Theory is all about. We'll make it as easy as pie to digest, minus the calories!
- **Get Active!**: Think you're not the 'exercise' type? Think again! I've got a mix of fun, quirky, and oh-so-easy exercises for you. From belting out your favorite tunes (shower acoustics recommended) to laughing your socks off (literally), there's something for everyone.
- **Bonus Brain Food**: Ever had a 'gut feeling'? Well, it's not just a figure of speech. We'll dive into the captivating tango between your belly and brain. Plus, for those parent-superheroes out there, I've got gems on how to nurture and protect your little one's Vagus Nerve.

NAVIGATING YOUR ULTIMATE VAGUS VOYAGE: THE BENEFITS & YOUR ROADMAP

By choosing this bundle, you've embarked on a transformative journey. Before you dive into the chapters, let's explore the benefits you stand to gain and a suggested plan to harness the full potential of this bundle.

Benefits You'll Reap:

- **Deep Understanding**: Get to know the Vagus Nerve and the Polyvagal Theory like they're your new BFFs. Knowledge is power, and you're about to be supercharged.
- **Emotional Mastery**: Gain tools to better regulate your emotions, say goodbye to unnecessary anxiety, and welcome tranquility into your life.
- **Health Boost**: By following the exercises, your body will thank you with improved well-being and perhaps even a springier step.
- **Child Care Gold**: For the caregivers, gain indispensable knowledge on nurturing a child's Vagus Nerve, setting them up for a healthier life.
- **Brain & Gut Synchrony**: Uncover the magic between your gut and brain, and understand those 'gut feelings' like never before.

YOUR ROADMAP TO MAXIMUM BENEFITS

- **Start Slow**: Begin with the "What is the Vagus Nerve?" and "What is the Polyvagal Theory?" chapters. Establishing a foundation will make the subsequent chapters even more enlightening.
- **Put It into Practice**: As you read about each exercise or technique, pause and try them out. Experience is the best teacher.
- **Journal It**: Keep a small diary to jot down observations, feelings, or changes you notice. This makes your journey interactive and personal.
- **Child Focus**: If you're a parent or caregiver, pay special attention to the chapter on "Healing Your Child's Vagus Nerve." It's golden information for the young ones.
- **Weekly Reviews**: At the end of each week, revisit your journal. Reflect on the exercises that felt good and those that didn't. It helps in tailoring a routine that suits you best.

- **Engage with Others**: Share tidbits with friends or family. Discussing your findings can offer new perspectives and make the journey more enriching.
- **End with Bonus**: Once you've gone through the main content, dive into the bonus chapters. They'll tie up any loose ends and offer additional insights.

SHARE YOUR HONEST FEEDBACK

We've journeyed through the intricacies of the Vagus Nerve and the Polyvagal Theory, and we hope it's been enlightening. However, no journey is complete without reflection, and we want to hear about your experiences.

Why? Because your feedback not only helps us understand your perspective but also aids in refining and improving future editions of this bundle. Whether it's a light bulb moment, a point of confusion, or something you felt was missing, we're all ears!

How to Leave Your Feedback:

- **Online Review**: Drop your thoughts on Amazon. These reviews guide future readers and provide a snapshot of varied experiences.
- **Direct Email**: We appreciate detailed feedback. Feel free to send us your thoughts, experiences, or suggestions at [author's email address].
- **Engage on Social Media**: Share your journey, insights, or critiques on our official social media platforms. Tag us so we can join the conversation!

Remember, every perspective is unique and offers a wealth of insights. Your honest feedback is like a compass, guiding us towards better and more impactful content.

INTRODUCTION

You've probably heard of the vagus nerve, but you might not know what it does. The vagus nerve is a complex, ancient structure. It is a major player in your body's autonomic nervous system, which controls your heart rate and blood pressure. The vagus nerve regulates digestion, breathing, blood pressure, heart rate, and several other functions in the body.

As a result of the number of functions the vagus nerve is responsible for, it is important that you know how to use yours effectively. However, as we get older, our vagus nerve can start to deteriorate - and this can cause problems like digestive issues and poor sleep quality. Fortunately for the human race, there are certain things that we could do to regenerate our vagus nerve and keep it functioning perfectly.

By understanding how the vagus nerve works, you can learn how to stimulate it with simple exercises like deep breathing or even blowing into a straw. These exercises can help you lower your blood pressure, improve your mood, and reduce stress levels. They are an excellent way to strengthen your vagus nerve and improve your overall health. In fact, they are even proven to help reverse the damage done by chronic stress.

To help keep your nerves healthy as you age, we recommend doing some simple exercises that stimulate your vagus nerve every day! And don't worry, they are very simple, practicable, and useful for all ages and gender, so you'll most likely be able to practice them alongside your friends and family.

Asides from vagus nerve exercises, we have also included extensive and well-detailed explanations about the workings of the vagus nerve, and by extension, the parasympathetic system. Be rest assured that everything you need to know about how to get your nervous system to relax and function at an optimum level is right within the pages of this book.

So without further ado, let's get started!

DAILY VAGUS NERVE EXERCISES

DAILY VAGUS NERVE EXERCISES

INTRODUCTION

INTRODUCTION

Our bodies are built to survive and live without conscious thinking. As we grow physically, our capacity for thinking grows exponentially. This is possible because our survival systems are regulated subconsciously or, more accurately, are automated. Our forebrains develop and enable our brains to process information, reflect, and interact with the world. In the meantime, our brainstems keep our bodies alive and healthy.

The brainstem is the densest and highest point of the spinal cord. It contains a variety of information control centers, or nuclei, each of which has particular tasks that they manage and signals that they send or receive.

Specific systems can alert us to internal stressors and threats to our survival within the natural environment. It doesn't matter if these stressors are an infection beginning to spread within bodies, worried thoughts about tasks to be completed, or our overall existence in our vicinity. The automatic actions of these systems enable us to endure.

The mechanisms that regulate these functions are controlled by a different branch of the autonomic system -the sympathetic branch, also known as the sympathetic nervous system. This system is responsible for boosting the heart rate, improving breath rate, reducing breathing depth, and shunting blood flow to muscles located in the legs and arms in a way that pulls blood away from the digestive tract and dilates our pupils. If the sympathetic nervous system becomes activated and in full swing, it is known as "the "fight-or-flight" state because this system helps us to either combat stressors or to "take flight" and run away from stressors.

There is another branch of the autonomic nervous system that lets us rest and recover from the stresses and responsibilities of our day. It helps us stay at peace, reduces heart and breathing rates, takes longer, more full breaths, and redirects blood flow away from our legs and internal organs. It lets our bodies recover in a calm and peaceful state and procreate. This part of the autonomic nervous system is called "parasympathetic." When the parasympathetic nervous system becomes active, it is known as "the "rest-and-digest" state.

The majority of the actions of the parasympathetic nervous system run through a particular pair of nerves within the body, known as the vagus nerve, which is the subject of this text. This nerve runs from the brainstem and traverses the entire body down to the abdomen. The vagus nerve controls the lungs, heart, and muscles of the throat and the airway, stomach, liver, pancreas, gallbladder, kidneys, spleen and small intestine, and a part of the large intestine.

The vagus nerve is the primary connection between the brain and the gut's microbiome, making it responsible for an extensive range of messages and signals around the body. This nerve is the primary communication route for nutrition, digestion, and the constantly changing number of viruses, bacteria, yeast, parasites, and worms living in our digestive tracts. For this reason, proper functioning of the vagus nerve is a significant indicator of good health, while vagus nerve dysfunction is the underlying reason for many diseases.

Harmony among all branches of the nervous system is essential to living a whole life. In essence, if there is an impediment to the function of one branch, instability and imbalance within the body ensue, ultimately leading to illness. For example, if stress levels stay overly high, the parasympathetic system will be unable to function optimally. It'll slowly lose the capacity to perform its duties, meaning that most bodily functions and blood flow will fall to the sympathetic branch.

Over time, blood circulation to the parasympathetic branch is likely to be restricted, and consequently, its function will diminish. In the same vein, overactivation of the parasympathetic system could reduce the ability of your body to handle the stressors that could be a threat to your life.

When we are constantly stressed, our bodies generate excessive levels of inflammation. We do not have the chance to rest and recuperate, which is necessary to ensure optimal performance. It is why we're breaking down more quickly and frequently than before. The risks of developing autoimmune disorders like rheumatoid arthritis, Hashimoto's thyroiditis, and multiple sclerosis are now higher than ever experienced in the medical system. Many people are experiencing all sorts of heart diseases and cancers, while diabetes and obesity are increasing alarmingly. In general, our overall nervous system has never looked so bad.

1

WHAT IS THE VAGUS NERVE?

The Vagus nerve is the key to unlocking the body's natural ability to heal itself.

WHAT IS THE VAGUS NERVE?

*A*t some point in your life, you may have encountered the term 'vagus nerve', probably on your favourite medical TV series or during a routine visit to the doctor. You should have paid the term more extreme attention and dismissed it as another medical jargon you should never understand. It might excite you to know that the vagus nerve is not half as complicated as you may have made it up to be.

This nerve is an essential member of the central nervous system (CNS) and is indispensable to the smooth running of the human body. From overseeing the digestion of that delicious meal you just had to slow down your heart rate and breathing as you fall asleep, the vagus nerve is a significant player in coordinating several bodily functions, and therefore, it deserves all the attention it can get from us.

The word 'vagus' is Latin, translating into 'wandering' or 'vagrant' in English. This term illustrates the course of the vagus nerve across the body and how this nerve interacts with all the organs in its path like a wanderer might. The vagus nerve is, in fact, the longest nerve in the body, running from the brain through the face and thorax to the abdomen.

The vagus nerve is a part of the cranial nerves, a set of 12 nerves in the back of the brain that send signals between the brain, face, neck, and torso. The vagus nerve is the tenth of the 12 cranial nerves and one of the most important members of this group. Before we move on, we will take a quick look at the other cranial nerves, as a knowledge of their functions might shed some light on the vagus nerve. They are:

1. **Olfactory nerve**: in charge of the sense of smell
2. **Optic nerve**: in the amount of sight
3. **Oculomotor nerve**: in charge of eye muscle motor function (movement) and pupil response to light
4. **Trochlear nerve**: in charge of the superior oblique muscle that controls the downward, outward, and inward movement of the eyes
5. **Trigeminal nerve**: in charge of facial sensations and the movement of jaw and ear muscles
6. **Abducens nerves**: in charge of the lateral rectus muscle, which controls outward and sideways eye movement
7. **Facial nerve**: in charge of facial expressions and sense of taste for some parts of the tongue
8. **Auditory/Vestibulocochlear nerve**: in charge of hearing and balance
9. **Glossopharyngeal nerve**: in charge of flavour at the back of the tongue and the ability to swallow
10. **Vagus Nerve**
11. **Accessory nerve**: in charge of the movement of the shoulder and neck muscles
12. **Hypoglossal nerve**: in charge of tongue movement.

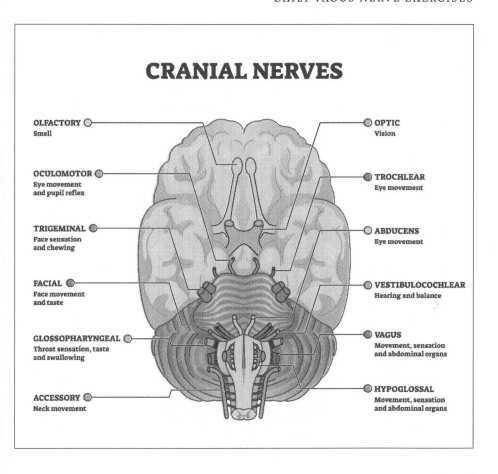

Image 1
Image Source: Kenhub.com

Seeing that all the cranial nerves mentioned above have peculiar functions allocated to them, one might begin to wonder, 'What is the function of the vagus nerve?' The vagus nerve is responsible for several functions, ranging from sending sensory information from the ear canal, throat, chest and trunk, as well as by allowing control of the muscles in your throat, compartment, and trunk, and finally, a sense of taste close to the root of your tongue.

The vagus nerve is one of the significant components of the parasympathetic (rest and digest) nervous system in the body's central nervous system, containing approximately 75% of the parasympathetic nerves. The parasympathetic nervous system controls all involuntary actions an individual performs, like brain function, heart rate and digestion.

The vagus nerve consists of two main sections: the right and left vagus nerves, which comprise motor and sensory nerve fibres with which they control motor (movement) and sensory functions. The motor component of the vagus nerve originates *from the basal plate of embryonic medulla oblongata* -a rounded mound at the end of the brain stem that connects with your spinal cord. On the other hand, the sensory component originates from the cranial neural crest, a group of migratory cells that give rise to various structures in the body.

The vagus nerve comprises approximately 80% afferent nerve fibres - nerve fibres responsible for carrying sensory information from the organs into the brain- and 20% efferent nerve fibres -responsible for transmitting data from the brain to the effector organs. This composition enables the vagus nerve to effectively retrieve and send information to and from the brain and organs.

ANATOMY AND COURSE OF THE VAGUS NERVE

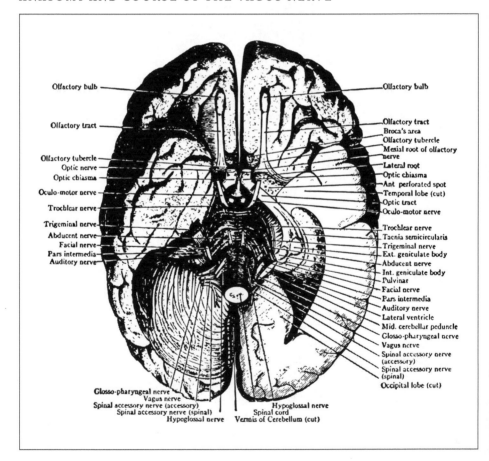

Immagine 1
Reiner hartmannpress

As seen in **Image 1** above, the vagus nerve has the longest course in the body, originating from the head and running across the thorax down to the abdomen. It also has the widest distribution, containing somatic and visceral afferent fibres and general and special visceral efferent fibres. This nerve originates and begins its course from the brain, developing from the fourth branchial arch, which is an embryologic structure that develops into anatomic structures in the adult human and is equally responsible for the development of other vital structures such as the pharyngeal and laryngeal muscles, the aortic arch and the subclavian artery.

The vagus nerve is divided **into the right** and **left vagus nerve.**

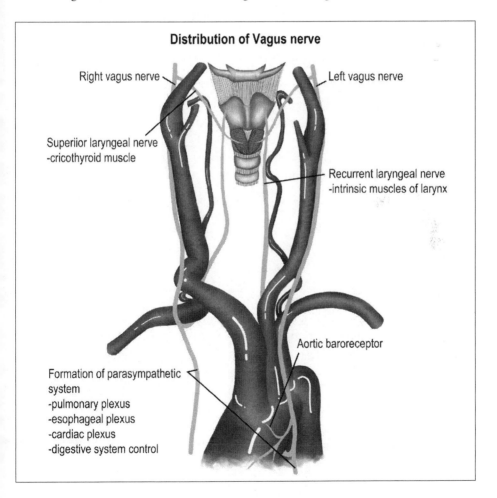

Distribution of Vagus nerve

Right vagus nerve

Left vagus nerve

Superiior laryngeal nerve
-cricothyroid muscle

Recurrent laryngeal nerve
-intrinsic muscles of larynx

Aortic baroreceptor

Formation of parasympathetic
system
-pulmonary plexus
-esophageal plexus
-cardiac plexus
-digestive system control

Immagine 2
Reiner hartmannpress

On leaving the brainstem's medulla oblongata, the right vagus nerve runs later-ally along the skull from the cranial or skull vault. Then it exits the head through the jugular foramen, a large opening at the base of the head. It then passes verti-cally *into the carotid sheath among the internal carotid artery and internal jugular up to the face and neck,* supplying sensory and motor innervation. It reaches the thorax and then moves behind the hilum of the right lung, which is a triangular section on the inner aspect of the lung that connects the lungs to their supporting structures. It is also where pulmonary vessels enter and exits your lungs. From here, it travels medially towards the oesophagus, which merges with the left vagus nerve to form the oesophageal plexus -a group of nerves supplying it.

On leaving the medulla oblongata, the **left vagus nerve** passes in front of the left subclavian artery to enter the thorax between the left common carotid and subclavian arteries. It runs down along the left side of the aortic arch, a part of the large vessel that carries blood from the heart to the organs. It then travels behind the phrenic nerve and changes course medially and downwards to reach the oesophageal hiatus, where it meets with the right vagus nerve to form the oesophageal plexus.

Passing through the oesophageal hiatus - an opening in the diaphragm through which the oesophagus passes into the abdominal cavity - the vagus nerve gains entry into the abdomen, where it contributes to the innervation of the viscera, down to the colon. The branches of the right vagus nerve form the posterior gastric plexus - a group of nerves that supply the stomach and intestines - on the rear surface of the stomach. In contrast, the branches of the left vagus nerve form the anterior gastric plexus on the anterior surface of the stomach.

Both plexuses course between the layers of the lesser omentum - a membrane that attaches the lesser curvature of the stomach to the liver superiority - with the fibres from the anterior gastric plexus running as far as the pylorus - the part of the stomach that connects it to the duodenum of the intestines and the upper part of the duodenum. The posterior vagal trunk and the posterior gastric branches send fibres to the significant abdominal autonomic plexus, a collection of parasym-pathetic and sympathetic nerve fibres that merge to innervate the organs and structures of the abdomen. From the plexus, vagal fibres are distributed to the territories of celiac, renal and superior mesenteric arteries.

Besides giving some output to several organs, the vagus nerve is between 80% and 90% of nerves, mainly conveying sensory information from the body's organs to the central nervous system.

In the brainstem's medulla oblongata, the vagus nerve also includes axons- thin nerve fibres responsible for transmitting impulses from one nerve cell to another. These axons originate from or merge onto four nuclei of the medulla. These axons include:

1. **The vagus' nerve dorsal nucleus**: It sends parasympathetic output to the viscera, particularly the intestines
2. **The nucleus is ambiguous**: It is a pair of nerve cells that *gives rise to the branchial efferent motor fibres of the vagus nerve and preganglionic parasympathetic neurons that* supply the heart.
3. **The solitary nucleus**: This nucleus receives afferent taste sensation from the tongue and primary afferent nerve fibres from visceral organs
4. **The spinal trigeminal nucleus**: It receives information about deep or crude touch, pain, and temperature of the external ear, the dura of the posterior cranial fossa, and the larynx mucosa.

Branches of the Vagus Nerve

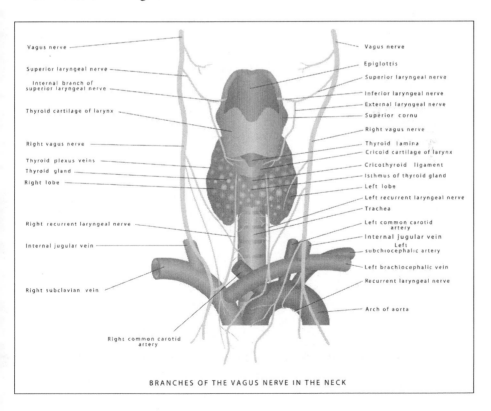

BRANCHES OF THE VAGUS NERVE IN THE NECK

Immagine 3
Reiner hartmannpress

Along its course from the brain to the abdomen, the vagus nerve gives out several innervating branches that supply sensory, motor and parasympathetic nerves to several organs and body parts. Here are the various departments that can be found in different parts of the body:

In the Head and the Neck

The branches of the vagus nerve that arise in the neck include:

1. **Meningeal branches**: It supplies the dura (the outermost membrane covering the brain and spinal cord) of the posterior cranial fossa
2. **Articular branches**: It innervates the external tympanic membrane, which is also known as the eardrum, and a small portion of the posterior part of the outer ear
3. **Pharyngeal branches**: These supply the muscles of the pharynx or throat
4. **Superior laryngeal branches**: It innervates the two cricothyroid muscles of the larynx or voice box
5. **Recurrent laryngeal branches**: That innervate all the intrinsic muscles of the larynx except the cricothyroid powers. It also supplies the oesophagus
6. **Superior cervical cardiac units**: They give off units to form the cardiac plexus
7. **Inferior cervical cardiac** components also give off branches to form the cardiac plexus.

In the Thorax

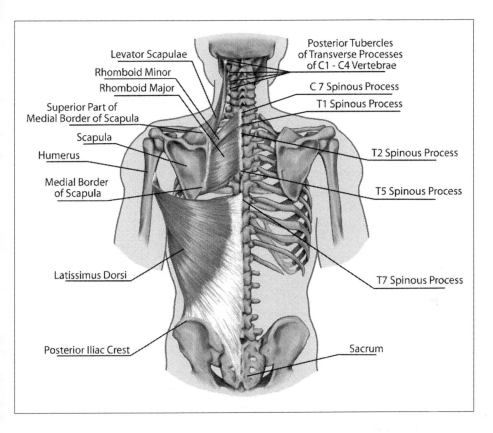

Immagine 4
Reiner hartmannpress

The branches of the vagus nerve that arise in the thorax include:

1. **Anterior vagal trunk**: It gives off branches to the oesophageal plexus, and it is made up of the following: Hepatic branch, Celiac branch, and Anterior gastric branches
2. **Posterior vagal trunk**: It also contributes to the oesophageal plexus, and it has two branches; the Celiac branch and the Posterior gastric branches
3. **Thoracic, cardiac units**: They give off extensions to form the cardiac plexus
4. Components of the **pulmonary plexus**

In the Abdomen
In the abdomen, the vagus nerve terminates and forms:

15

1. **The anterior gastric plexus**: This plexus provides innervation to the stomach
2. **The posterior gastric plexus**: It innervates the rear surface of the stomach, and its terminal branches are known as "crow's foot", which supply the [pyloric antrum] and the posterior wall of the pyloric canal.

Functions of the Vagus Nerve

The vagus nerve oversees numerous aspects and functions in the human body, most of which are actions we have no control over. Hence, the importance of the vagus nerve in the body should be emphasized. Some of the functions in the different parts of the body include:

In the Head and Neck

The vagus nerve has motor and sensory functions in the head region. Its sensory functions include:

1. The vagus nerve is responsible for taste sensation from the posterior two-thirds of the mouth, including the upper third of the oesophagus.
2. The vagus nerve also carries sensory information from the skin behind the ear, the outer part of the ear canal.

In the head and neck, the vagus nerve regulates the motor functions of muscles of the neck, the pharynx, and intrinsic muscles of the larynx (except the cricothyroid forces). These muscles are responsible for speech, probation and swallowing.

In the Thorax

The vagus nerve branches supply parasympathetic nerves to most organs occupying the chest region. It plays a significant role in overseeing the various functions of these organs necessary to living, such as sweating, breathing, reflexes like sneezing, coughing, gag reflex, etc. These organs include:

1. **The trachea**: The trachea is one of the structures involved in breathing. Hence, the vagus nerve plays a role in maintaining a smooth breathing process, reflexes like sneezing, coughing, gag reflex, etc.
2. **The lower two-thirds of the oesophagus**: The vagus nerve is essential for reflex relaxation of the lower oesophagal sphincter, which are ring-like muscles that close and open to control the movement of substances into the stomach. This is to allow swallowing.
3. **The lungs**: The vagus nerve is crucial in regulating airflow in the lungs, cough reflex as well as mucus secretion

4. **The heart**: In the cardiovascular system, the vagus nerve plays a vital role in regulating and maintaining heart rate and blood pressure.

In the Abdomen

The abdominal branches of the vagus nerve also provide parasympathetic innervation to the organs in the abdomen and play a vital role in the smooth running of involuntary actions like peristalsis and digestion, hormonal secretion, hunger and satiety. These organs include:

1. **The stomach**: In the stomach, the vagus nerve is a significant player in promoting digestion. It achieves this by facilitating peristalsis - the movement of food substances and gastric emptying of food bolus into the intestines.
2. **The liver**: In the liver, the vagus nerve has an essential role in the maintenance and regulation of glucose production (gluconeogenesis)
3. **The intestines**: In the intestines, the vagus nerve aids digestion by sending signals to the brain, transforming the microflora or bacteria in the intestine into those necessary for digestion.

2

THE VAGUS NERVE AND THE PARASYMPATHETIC NERVOUS SYSTEM

The Vagus nerve is the conductor of the body's symphony of health and well-being.

THE VAGUS NERVE AND THE PARASYMPATHETIC NERVOUS SYSTEM

*H*ave you ever considered how your body can smoothly interact with your surroundings, respond appropriately to specific situations and not miss a beat? Well, all these actions are possible because of an intricate system called the nervous system. The nervous system is involved in virtually everything an individual does, from falling asleep and staying asleep, waking up, breathing, eating and responding to stressful and threatening situations to growing, ageing, and even flashing a beautiful smile when happy. Simply put, the range of activities the nervous system covers is limitless.

Due to the system's complexity, it has been grouped into two divisions for detailed understanding and study. The divisions are:

- **The Central Nervous System**: this encompasses the brain and the spinal cord and
- **The Peripheral Nervous System** encompasses all afferent and efferent nerves that relay information from the brain and spinal cord to all the peripheral organs and structures.

While the central nervous system has no further divisions, the peripheral nervous system is divided into the somatic and autonomic nervous systems. The jumpy bodily system regulates all voluntary muscular systems within the body; the process of voluntary reflex arcs and processes sensory information that arrives via external stimuli, including sight, hearing and touch. On the other hand, the autonomic nervous system is responsible for regulating unconscious and involuntary bodily processes. These processes include heart rate and rhythm, blood flow, respiratory rate and breathing, pupillary response, urination, flight or fight response, sexual arousal and digestion.

Once again, the autonomic nervous system is subdivided into the sympathetic and parasympathetic systems. However, some schools of thought add a third system - the enteric nervous system - to this classification. The sympathetic nervous system is well-known as the "fight or flight" system, while the parasympathetic nervous system is often deemed the "rest and digest" or "feed and breed" system.

Here is an image that better explains the breakdown of the nervous system:

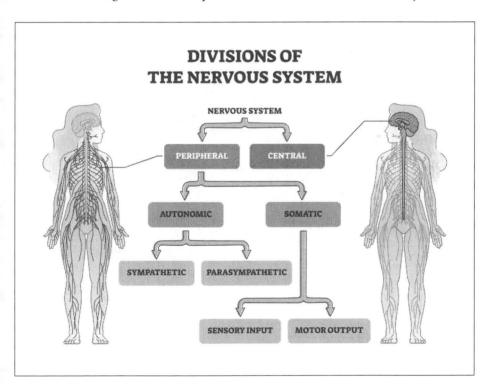

DIVISIONS OF
THE NERVOUS SYSTEM

NERVOUS SYSTEM

PERIPHERAL | CENTRAL

AUTONOMIC | SOMATIC

SYMPATHETIC | PARASYMPATHETIC

SENSORY INPUT | MOTOR OUTPUT

Immagine 5
Reiner hartmannpress

The vagus nerve is *the most important nerve of the parasympathetic system*, thus making it our primary concern in this chapter to establish the relationship between the two. To fully understand the vagus nerve's role in the parasympathetic nervous system, one must first understand the scope of functions the parasympathetic system performs.

Above, it has been stated that the autonomic system oversees the regulation of involuntary actions, and the parasympathetic 'rest and digest' division of this system controls involuntary movements that occur when the body is at rest, especially after eating. These activities include sexual arousal, salivation, lacrimation, urination, digestion and defecation.

Facilitating most of these functions is the vagus nerve. Dr Stephen Porges, a University Scientist at Indiana University and author of The Polyvagal Theory, says in his book about understanding the nervous system and how the tone of the vagus nerve directly affects our wellness - "The brain is reading and regulating your body through this nerve ... The body won't function optimally unless it (the vagus nerve) picks up safety cues." This shows the significant yet complex relationship between the vagus nerve and the parasympathetic system.

Up to now, scientists are still discovering new processes and connections between these two components. However, here is a breakdown of how the vagus nerve relates to the parasympathetic system in the body: Edit from here.

In the Cardiovascular System

The vagus nerve plays a fundamental role in maintaining physiological homeostasis (the normal healthy state necessary for survival) in the heart and circulatory system. The vagal branches: superior and inferior cervical and thoracic cardiac branches combine with cardiac branches of the sympathetic nerves to form the cardiac nerve plexus that innervates the heart.

Electrical impulses travel from the heart via the efferent nerve fibres to the nucleus, ambiguous in the brainstem. In a healthy heart, the sinoatrial node is the central pacemaker or generator of electric impulses. The sinoatrial node is mainly responsible for the cardiac cell automaticity, or rather the ability of the cells to generate electrical activity free of external stimulation. The electrical impulse naturally produced by the sinoatrial node sets the pace for the other electrical fibres like the atrioventricular node and the bundle of it and the rest of the heart.

When a healthy individual is awake, the SA node typically maintains a heart rate between 60 to 100 beats per minute. When you sleep or are in a condition where the heart is tachycardic - beating too fast, like in stressful situations, the vagus nerve is stimulated, resulting in an overall decrease in the heart rate and blood pressure.

The vagus afferent nerves receive information from the brain, relay it to the heart and then act on the sinoatrial node, slowing its conduction and modulating vagal tone through the help of the neurotransmitter acetylcholine. Neurotransmitters are chemical substances that tell cells what to do. The vagus nerve also stimulates a decrease in sodium and calcium ions influx into the cardiac cells.

Therefore, it contrasts the effect of the sympathetic nervous system resulting in reductions in heart rate, vascular resistance and arterial blood pressure.

In the Respiratory System

The vagus nerve's role should be emphasized, as it controls a myriad of activities in the overall smooth functioning of the lungs. Stimulation of the vagus nerve is placed in a constriction of the smooth muscle that lines the bronchi and bronchioles, a decrease in airway tone, and an increase in glandular secretions. This is due to the release of acetylcholine, which activates M3 muscarinic receptors (unique protein structures on cells and organs that receive and interpret stimulus) on airway smooth muscle to stimulate contraction.

The vagus nerve also mediates reflexes like coughing and the ability of the lungs to control the levels of oxygen and carbon dioxide. When you inhale dust, smoke, or pollen, or if food particles and liquid get into your trachea, your respiratory tract becomes irritated. The body tries to prevent the foreign body from gaining access to your lungs by eliciting the cough reflex. The cough receptors are stimulated, resulting in impulse transmission through the laryngeal nerve, a branch of the laryngeal nerve which arises from the vagus nerve to the nucleus tractus of the medulla - a pair of nerve cells found in the brainstem.

Following this, efferent responses are generated and transmitted to the organs involved in the cough reflex. The following events occur:

1. **Irritation** of cough receptors causes the vocal cords to open widely hence, allowing the entry of air into the lungs
2. **The diaphragm** and external intercostal muscles contract, with the diaphragm becoming flat. This increases the thoracic cavity space, facilitating air movement into the lungs and increasing pressure within the thorax.
3. **The epiglottis,** which is the covering of the trachea, and vocal cords close, trapping the air within the lungs
4. **The internal** intercostal and abdominal muscles contract to reduce the thoracic cavity. The vocal cords return to their anatomic state, and the

epiglottis opens. This releases the pressure from the lungs and causes both the air and the irritant to be rapidly removed.

During rest or sleep, the vagus nerve understands the signs of safety; it transmits these impulses via the afferent nerve endings of the vagus nerve to the brain, which in turn communicates with the diaphragm. This contributes to relaxation as the respiratory rate gradually reduces as you breathe deeply. This is one of the reasons why deep breathing is a way to activate the vagus nerve.

In the Digestive System

The vagus nerve is vital in facilitating digestion - both directly and indirectly. Even before you start eating, the vagus nerve is stimulated and begins producing acetylcholine which promotes gastric secretion. When food bolus enters the stomach, this enables the afferent nerve endings of the vagus nerve and generates sensory impulses.

Sensory fibres of the vagus transmit these sensory impulses to the sensory nucleus of the vagus, placed in the medulla of the brain stem. This nucleus, in turn, sends afferent impulses through the motor fibres of the vagus back to the stomach and causes the secretion of gastric juice, stimulation of smooth muscle contraction and relaxation of sphincters.

On entry of chyme into the intestines, the vagus nerve is stimulated, and this results in constriction of the intestinal smooth muscles and increased movement of food down the intestines. The vagus nerve also stimulates the production of digestive enzymes and hormones from organs like the liver and pancreas to indirectly facilitate digestion.

Gut-Brain Axis

In the last decades, scientists have made groundbreaking headway in understanding the complex relationship between the microflora, the gut and the brain. This relationship involves exchanging information between the brain and the heart via the vagus nerve, as it can sense the presence of gut microorganisms and send relevant feedback to the brain. The gut contains millions of microorganisms that produce chemicals that drive the digestion of food by sending impulses through the vagus nerve to the brain to increase the production of digestive enzymes.

Scientists have also discovered that these microorganisms produce the neurotransmitter gamma-aminobutyric acid (GABA), which helps control feelings of fear and anxiety. This is why you probably feel your stomach drop when something negative happens or you are very anxious. Hence, the gut-brain axis also serves a cautionary or protective function.

In the Uro-Genital System

The ability of an individual to pass urine is a testimony to the operational coordination between the sympathetic and parasympathetic systems of our autonomic nervous system. When the bladder is full, afferent nerve fibres convey this information to the brain, and the brain responds by centrally increasing parasympathetic tone and decreasing sympathetic activity. This results in the relaxation of the internal sphincter muscle and a contraction of the bladder. The vagus nerve, being the 'queen nerve' of the parasympathetic system, also controls the muscle contraction of the bladder during urination.

Apart from urination, the parasympathetic system, especially the pudendal nerve- an important nerve of the pelvis originating from S2-S4 and the vagus nerve also plays a vital role in achieving sexual arousal as it is one of the excitatory pathways by which an individual is aroused. During arousal, excitatory signals can emanate in the brain, either by the sight or the thought of a desirable sexual partner or by physical genital stimulation. Independent of the source of these signals generated, these signals are transmitted to the excitatory nerves in the penis, and they respond by releasing pro-erectile neurotransmitters like nitric oxide and acetylcholine. These kinds of chemical messengers signal the smooth muscles of the penile arteries to control and fill with blood, resulting in male erections, or they result in stimulation of the glands in the vagina to produce lubricating fluid.

The vagus nerve also promotes *sexual arousal indirectly via endocrine or hormonal pathways by stimulating sex hormones like testosterone and estrogen.*

Hormone Expression

Hormones are an integral aspect of the human body as these hormones regulate growth, sex drive, sexual development, reproduction, sexual function, metabolism, etc. The parasympathetic system, particularly the vagus nerve stimulation, is essential to the elaboration of hormones required for the full functioning of the body. Some hormones released include oxytocin, testosterone, and vasoactive intestinal peptide. The production of growth hormone-releasing hormone and the activation of parathyroid hormone for converting vitamin D3 to active vitamin D also rely on the vagus Nerve.

In the Immune System

Vagal nerve stimulation has been implicated in parasympathetic control of physiological homeostasis, immune defence mechanisms, inflammatory reflexes and process reduction. It has been discovered that inflammation, which is the body's method of fighting against harmful things, such as infections, injuries, and toxins, in an attempt to heal itself, is the primary trigger for most chronic diseases, such as diabetes mellitus and Alzheimer's disease.

In most chronic diseases, the body cannot recognize its cells. Instead, it tags them as foreign and destroys them, and low vagal tone has been associated with chronic or prolonged inflammation. Research has also shown that individuals with inflammatory disorders, like rheumatoid arthritis and other autoimmune diseases, frequently have diminished heart rate variability, a marker of reduced vagal tone.

This reduced vagal tone activates the production of proinflammatory cytokines, which are substances secreted by inflammatory cells. These cytokines can influence other cells' activities and increase sympathetic nervous system activity and stress hormones by contributing to systemic inflammation.

In the inflammatory reflex, the activity of afferent vagus nerve fibres in the nodose ganglion is stimulated by cytokines and pathogen-associated molecular patterns. The impulses generated are transmitted to the nucleus tractus solitaries, and mutual connections between the nucleus tractus solitaries - a collection of solely sensory nerve cell bodies in the medulla oblongata, and the default mode network- mediate communication and activation of efferent vagus nerve fibres from the default mode network.

The signal is transmitted to the celiac ganglia, which is a collection of nerves that supply: the inferior part of the oesophagus, stomach, pancreas, spleen, kidneys, liver, gallbladder, and small intestine as it is also transmitted to the superior mesenteric ganglion in the celiac plexus, where the splenic nerve originates. Norepinephrine released from the splenic nerve binds to β2-adrenergic receptors and causes the release of acetylcholine from T cells (immune system cells that fight infections), containing functional choline acetyltransferase.

Acetylcholine then binds to nicotinic acetylcholine receptors on macrophages, specialized cells detecting and destroying bacteria and other harmful organisms. This interaction suppresses proinflammatory cytokine release from these cells and inflammation. Vagal nerve stimulation also improves survival in sepsis, hemor-rhagic shock, and ischemia-reperfusion injury, which is tissue damage because of the blood return supply to tissue after a period of lack of oxygen or oxygenated blood.

Vagus nerve and splenic nerve signalling mediated through nicotinic acetyl-choline receptors on splenocytes - a type of white blood cell, controls inflamma-tion in acute kidney injury and alleviates the condition. Hence, vagal nerve stimulation also provides defensive actions against liver injury caused by inhibiting oxidative stress and apoptosis or cell self-destruction, decreasing inflammatory cytokines and enhancing antioxidative capability in the liver.

In Social interaction

In social gatherings, the vagus nerve encourages individuals to be friendly and agreeable, or what Stephen Porges, a University Scientist at Indiana University, calls the "compassionate witness,". It is a physiological state where an individual is not emitting cues of anger, threat or hurt; however, it is there as a serene and supportive observer. *"The co-regulation helps the nervous system of those who have been hurt to feel safe enough without being defensive, to feel calm"*, *Porges* says.

3

VAGUS NERVE DISORDERS

The Vagus nerve is the bridge between the mind and the body, connecting us to our emotions and physical sensations.

VAGUS NERVE DISORDERS

*V*agus nerve derangements may occur in overactivity or under-activity of vagal functions. When the nerve is under-activity, the resultant disorder is gastroparesis, while overactivity causes vasovagal syncope. Vagus nerve abnormalities have also been implicated in certain lung disorders, such as chronic obstructive pulmonary disease, lung fibrosis, and lung cancer. Let's take a look at the most common vagus nerve disorders.

Gastroparesis

Gastroparesis, also well-known as delayed gastric emptying, is a medical condition affecting the stomach's normal motility. It is characteristic of weak muscular contractions or stomach peristalsis, resulting in food and liquid retention in the stomach for a prolonged period. Food and other stomach contents leave the stomach more slowly into the duodenum of the intestines. This could result in consistent nutrient absorption, adequate nutrition and better glycemic control.

One of the most typical causes of this disease is autonomic neuropathy or nerve damage, especially damage to the vagus nerve. This may occur in individuals with longstanding chronic diseases like type 1 or type 2 diabetes, as high blood glucose levels may cause chemical changes in the nerve. The vagus nerve thus becomes damaged by years of high blood glucose or insufficient glucose transport into cells resulting in gastroparesis.

Due to the loss of vagal stimulation and acetylcholine release, the gastric cells fail to release nitric oxide. Thus, when nitric oxide levels are low, smooth muscle function and other organs essential to digestion may not function optimally. The loss of vagal stimulation may also affect other vital components of the stomach, such as the interstitial cells of Cajal.

The interstitial cells of Cajal act as a pacemaker in the gastric smooth muscles as they transduce signals from motor neurons to generate electrical impulses and rhythm in the smooth muscle cells. Lower nitric oxide levels are also associated with the loss of these cells, which could eventually result in the loss of function of the smooth muscles in the stomach and other areas of the gastrointestinal tract.

It has been discovered that gastroparesis tends to affect the female gender more than the males, and some schools of thought also believe that gastroparesis symptoms tend to worsen the week before menstruation when progesterone levels are highest.

Certain factors can also predispose an individual to gastroparesis. However, it is not a guarantee that individuals with any of these factors would have gastroparesis, the likelihood of developing the disease is higher:

- Diabetes
- Abdominal or esophageal surgery
- Infection, typically viral infections.
- Cigarette smoking
- Advanced age, usually from the 4th decade of life
- Certain medications able to slow the rate of stomach emptying, like narcotic pain pills
- Scleroderma — a connective tissue disease
- Nervous system diseases, like Parkinson's disease or multiple sclerosis
- Thyroid gland derangement, such as hypothyroidism, decreases thyroid function.

Signs and Symptoms of Gastroparesis

Gastroparesis is associated with many signs and symptoms, some of which are diagnostic. For this reason, assisting the physician to diagnose without resorting to invasive investigative methods. Some of these signs and symptoms include:

- Persistent nausea

- Abdominal pain
- Vomiting, particularly undigested food
- Early satiety or feeling full after consuming a few morsels of food
- Abdominal bloating
- Heartburn
- Gastroesophageal Acid reflux (GERD)
- Body aches
- Abnormal blood glucose levels
- Lack of appetite
- Morning nausea
- Night sweats
- Palpitations
- Spasms of the stomach wall
- Constipation or infrequent bowel movements
- Weight loss and malnutrition
- Muscle weakness and wasting
- Difficulty in swallowing.

Complications of Gastroparesis

Gastroparesis is associated with several complications arising from its aetiology and how the disease affects other organs in the body.

Abnormal Fluctuations in Blood Glucose Levels

Due to impaired motility and absorption in the digestive system, the rate at which glucose is absorbed is erratic. A high glucose meal retained in the stomach may be absorbed slowly for a very long time hence, keeping a steady stream of glucose into the blood and aggravating diabetes if present.

Severe Dehydration

Gastroparesis could cause severe and possibly life-threatening dehydration in patients due to impaired absorption of fluid and the vomiting associated with the disease. The individual's digestive system fails to optimally absorb the liquid and electrolytes required to maintain blood level at the homeostatic range and keep other physiological processes running. They are also losing the little that is being absorbed by vomiting. Hence, if not managed immediately, dehydration in gastroparesis may further compound problems and lead to more severe complications such as dizziness, seizures and shock.

Bowel Obstruction

In gastroparesis, food slowly moves to the intestines, causing a build-up. The longer food remains without being digested, the more fluid is drawn out, and as fluid is drawn out, the food hardens and bezoars -solid masses of undigested food are formed. Over time, the intestines may become blocked by preventing the normal movement of the products of digestion.

Infections

Due to the prolonged retention of undigested food in the intestines in individuals with gastroparesis, an overgrowth of bacteria may ensue. This could further result in bacterial infections in the gut, especially in the small intestines.

Malnutrition

Malnutrition is a common complication of gastroparesis, as the digestive system cannot absorb nutrients optimally. Nutrients such as proteins, vitamins, etc., required for proper growth and functioning of bodily activities are not absorbed into the body. Moreover, the organs do not function properly, and the individual begins to lose weight and looks generally unhealthy without proper management.

Fatigue and General Body Weakness

As a result of the malnutrition associated with gastroparesis, individuals frequently complain of tiredness and general weakness. This is due to inadequate calorie and nutrient availability needed for daily activities.

Reduced Quality of Life

As a result of the associated symptoms and complications of gastroparesis, the individual may find it challenging to keep up with their daily activities and responsibilities. The individual may only be able to do what they enjoy with proper disease management freely.

Vasovagal Syncope

Vasovagal syncope, also known as reflex or neurocardiogenic syncope, is the most common type affecting individuals today, accounting for more than 50% of all cases. It is a medical condition that occurs because of the overactivity of the vagus nerve, characterized by a loss of consciousness due to a neurologically induced decrease in blood pressure and a decline in heart rate. Vasovagal syncope occurs typically following a stressful trigger, such as seeing blood, pain, hunger, fear, emotional stress, heat exposure, or prolonged standing.

As discussed earlier, the vagus nerve is physiologically responsible for decreasing heart rate, especially during relaxation or sleep. However, when the vagus nerve is abnormal, it interprets stimulus excessively and sends exaggerated impulses to the brain. The brainstem's nucleus tractus solitarii is then activated directly or indirectly by the triggering stimulation, resulting in concurrent enhancement of vagal tone and function in the heart and withdrawal of sympathetic nervous system tone. This, in turn, dramatically slows the heart rate and dilation of blood vessels, resulting in low blood pressure and, thus, insufficient blood flow to the brain.

Signs and Symptoms of Vasovagal Syncope

Depending on the degree of damage, vasovagal syncope presents various signs and symptoms of varying degrees. These symptoms may last between a few seconds to several minutes. Some of these signs and symptoms include:

1. Lightheadedness
2. Loss of consciousness
3. Nausea
4. Ringing in the ears
5. Pale skin
6. A feeling of extreme hot or cold, usually accompanied by sweating
7. An uneasy feeling in the heart
8. Confusion and unclear thought processes
9. A slight inability to speak correctly or form words, occasionally accompanied by mild stuttering
10. Weakness
11. Visual disturbances such as photophobia, blurred or tunnel vision, black spots in vision,
12. Nervousness or anxiety.

During a vasovagal syncope episode, you may notice the following in a generic individual:

1. Convulsive, unnatural movements
2. Slow, weak pulse and
3. Dilated pupils.

Complications of Vasovagal Syncope

- Reduced quality of life
- Injuries resulting from a fall when the individual loses consciousness
- It has been documented that recurrent syncope episodes may lead to short-term memory impairment due to decreased blood flow to the brain.

Lung Disorders

Research has shown that the vagus nerve has also been implicated in various pulmonary disorders, like asthma, chronic obstructive pulmonary condition (COPD), pulmonary fibrosis, acute respiratory distress syndrome (ARDS), and lung cancers. In chronic obstructive pulmonary disease, vagal nerve overactivity or dysregulation can lead to an increased sensitivity of the cough reflex such that the individual coughs exaggeratedly and inappropriately. Vagal dysregulation can also lead to increased activity of the parasympathetic reflex control of the airways, contributing to increased mucus secretion and bronchial smooth muscle contraction.

4

VAGUS NERVE EXERCISES

The Vagus nerve is the body's built-in stress relief system, and activating it can help reduce anxiety and depression.

*H*aving understood the importance of the vagus nerve and the role it plays in the day-to-day functioning of the human body, and having seen that this nerve is prone to dysfunction, this chapter and subsequent ones will explore the different ways through which the vagal nerve can be cared for to ensure that it functions as it should and vagal tone is optimal.

Vagal tone is an internal biological process indicating the vagal nerve's activities. In simple terms, the vagal tone is a determinant of the functionality of the vagus nerve. A high vagal tone indicates that the vagus nerve is functioning optimally, while a low vagal tone suggests that the vagus nerve is not working as it should. However, there are specific steps that an individual could take to prevent a vagal nerve dysfunction, the consequences of which have been discussed above or to improve vagal tone. Top on that list is vagal nerve exercises.

Vagus nerve exercises are physical and mental activities that enhance or maintain the vagus nerve's overall performance. Studies have shown that vagal nerve exercises are one of the most effective methods of stimulating the vagus nerve and increasing its functionality. Since these exercises aim to enhance and maintain the vagal nerve, they are suitable for individuals with low vagal tones and those with faultless vagal techniques. To determine which category you fall into and ascertain the functionality of your vagus nerve, you need to carry out a vagal tone test.

How To Do a Vagal Tone Test

Vagal tone tests are encouraged because they show vagal nerve functionality, indicate the kind of vagus nerve stimulation needed, and ultimately prevent the adverse consequences of vagal nerve dysfunction. While involving a health practitioner in a vagal nerve test is generally better, some tests can be carried out without medical supervision or knowledge. Let's take a look at the different types of vagal tone tests.

Gag Reflex Check

When conducting a gag reflex check to determine vagus nerve function, you would need help from a second party, either a doctor or a non-professional. Your partner could use a cotton swab to lightly prod at either side of the back of your throat. Your reaction to this should be a gag. If you do not, however, this could result from a vagal nerve problem.

If an individual does not gag, however, it could indicate a vagal nerve problem, further pointing toward a concern with brainstem function. When this occurs, vagus nerve stimulation is necessary to improve vagus nerve functioning.

However, in specific individuals, a vagus nerve dysfunction might not be the sole reason behind the absence of the gag reflex. Even though gagging is a regular neuromuscular action, you may have never experienced it because the areas in your mouth that could trigger gagging are less sensitive to physical touch. This is usually nothing to worry about. However, more extreme reasons include:

- Unilateral damage to the glossopharyngeal nerve
- Unilateral damage to the vagus nerve
- Brain death

Cardiovagal Tone Check

Research has shown that damage to the vagal nerve could result in complications of the cardiovascular system. As a result, an assessment of the cardiovascular system might provide clues as to the state of the vagus nerve. A doctor might carry out this test by measuring blood pressure, heart rate response, heart rate variability, heart rate changes due to the activation or obstruction of specific sensory nerves, and heart rate recovery after exercise, also known as parasympathetic reactivation.

The results of these measurements could shed some light on vagal nerve performance concerning the cardiovascular system and the general state of cardiovascular health.

Throat Check

The throat serves as one of the areas where the vagus nerve is distributed and, as a result, can be checked to determine vagal function. To carry out this test, you might need the help of a partner. You would have to open your mouth wide and have your partner look into your mouth, towards the back of your throat, in search of the uvula, the soft tissue flap that extends from the soft palate drops down at the back of the mouth.

To make your uvula and soft palate more accessible, you can use a finger or a tongue depressor to push your tongue down and a flashlight to light up the back of your mouth. Next, you should make an 'ah ah' sound and have your partner observe the position of your uvula.

If there is any deviation of the uvula, that is, any shift in position from one side to the other, it could be an indication of vagal nerve dysfunction. This dysfunction can be further classified by a medical expert based on the positioning of the uvula.

CT Scan or MRI

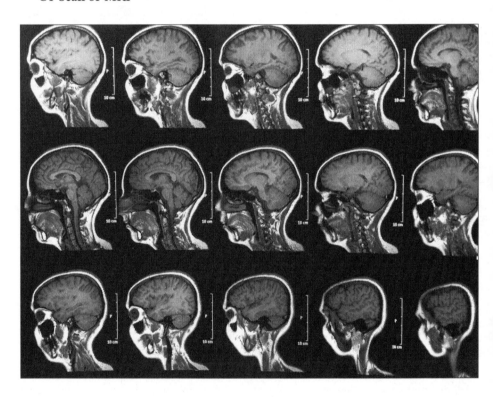

Immagine 6
Reiner hartmannpress

It has been reiterated throughout this book that the vagus nerve is the most important nerve of the parasympathetic system, which is responsible for several body functions, including digestion, heart rate, urination, and energy conservation. As a result, a problem with either of these functions could signify a problem with the vagus nerve, which provides another way to test the vagus nerve's tone.

While the gastrointestinal tract has some intrinsic nerves that provide it with substantial independent control over gastrointestinal functions, the central nervous system is still needed to provide external nerve inputs to moderate, balance, and unite these functions to produce desired results. This nerve provides parasympathetic innervation to the gastrointestinal tract and coordinates specific complex interactions.

If the functioning and control of the gastrointestinal tract are not top-notch, several gastrointestinal complications could arise, including chronic constipation, faecal impaction, bowel obstruction, and chronic diarrhoea. While some of these complications could result from other factors, some of them, such as intestinal blockages, can also be caused by a vagus nerve dysfunction. As such, a doctor could use a computed tomography (CT), magnetic resonance imaging (MRI) to look for intestinal blockages that could point toward a problem with the vagus nerve.

Gastric Emptying Solid Study

A gastric emptying study gauges how long food takes to move through the stomach and into the intestines. This test is carried out via an electronic device that will be ingested with the meal, allowing images of the stomach to be taken at various timed intervals.

Since the vagus nerve is responsible for digestion and ultimately controls the speed at which food is digested, a gastric emptying study can detect its state and functionalism. If the study shows that the digestion rate is slower or faster than usual, that could indicate a vagus nerve dysfunction.

Benefits of Vagus Nerve Exercises

If any of the vagus nerve functionality tests above indicate a vagus nerve dysfunction, then there is a need for exercises to stimulate the vagus nerve. The benefits of these exercises are vast and cannot be overemphasized. If you start carrying out vagus nerve exercises, it might be good to know their effects to recognize them when you feel them in your body.

Relieve Stress and Anxiety

Studies have shown that specific vagus nerve exercises could help relieve anxiety and chronic stress. This is not only because these exercises generally contain slow and relaxing movement patterns that can put the body in a state of calm but also because they stimulate the vagus nerve to trick and convince the brain that everything is okay, thus leading to relaxation.

One exercise that comes to mind is yoga, which contains a series of physical activities targeted at physical and mental wellness. Practising yoga or similar training during a period of heightened stress or anxiety can be very stimulating for your vagus nerve, thus resulting in a literal chill-out.

These exercises do not have to be done only when you feel stressed; practising them daily, even when you do not think you are stressed, is a great way to build resistance against stress. Health educator D'Elia Assenza says, "I believe we should prioritize our stress every day—even when we don't feel like we're stressed. It's a huge part of having optimal health".

Pain Relieve

One of the most beautiful things about the human mind is its inability to process more than one thing at a time. This implies that you are automatically distracted from others if you focus on one thing. Because of this, breathing exercises are one way a person can learn to shift their focus away from pain. This is especially so because many unknowingly practise breath holding or seizure while anticipating pain, thus activating the fight/flight response and increasing the pain sensation.

Aside from breathing exercises, other exercises equally stimulating the vagus nerve could help reduce pain if appropriately practised.

Treatment of Epilepsy

Vagus nerve stimulation through exercises has been proven effective in treating certain neurological conditions, including epilepsy. When used alongside anti-epileptic medications, vagus nerve stimulation could reduce the occurrence of abnormal electrical brain activities that result in seizures. A reduction of this sort could help slow down the frequency of these seizures and their severity and length.

Aside from dealing with seizures, vagus nerve exercises could also help an epileptic's post-seizure health, including recovery, cognition, mood and overall health.

Boosting Immunity and Overall Health

Vagus nerve stimulation through exercises can help to increase a person's immune system, thus helping them to ward off illnesses and lead healthier lives. Vagus nerve exercises help people with high blood pressure, or fast heart rates lower these rates and reduce the risk of cardiovascular occurrences such as strokes or heart attacks.

Studies have also shown that vagus nerve stimulation is effective in treating inflammation. This makes it great for people suffering from the following conditions:

- Rheumatoid arthritis
- Crohn's disease

- Inflammatory bowel disease
- Ulcerative colitis

Treatment of Mental Health Disorders

Research has shown that about 13% of the world's population suffers from mental health disorders, a figure steadily rising due to the effects of the Covid-19 pandemic. These mental disorders include schizophrenia, depression, bipolar disorders and post-traumatic stress disorder (PTSD).

Stimulation of the vagus nerve via exercises may positively affect a person's mental health, thus alleviating depression and other symptoms. It could also regulate a person's mood and emotions, helping them to replace feelings of panic and fear with calmness and clear-headedness.

5

DEEP AND SLOW BREATHING

The Vagus nerve is the body's innate healing mechanism, helping us to recover from trauma and injury.

DEEP AND SLOW BREATHING

*B*reathing has always been known to be essential to survival. It involves moving air into and from the lungs to facilitate the exchange of oxygen and carbon dioxide within the internal environment. For many years now, however, breathing has been discovered to be more than just respiration. Science has developed different breathing techniques that could facilitate various moods, including calm, relaxation, focus, pain relief, stress relief, and even sleep. Deep and slow breathing is another exercise that increases the parasympathetic system by stimulating the vagus nerve.

There are specific neurons located in the heart and the neck called baroreceptors. The function of these neurons is to detect blood pressure and then convey the neuronal signal to the brain. If these neurons see that a person's blood pressure is high, the signals they send to the brain will activate the vagus nerve to lower blood pressure and heart rate. This means that the person's sympathetic (fight or flight) system's activity reduces, and instead, there is an increase in the parasympathetic (rest and digest) system.

While these baroreceptors are generally sensitive, their sensitivity varies from person to person. And so, while one person's baroreceptors might take longer to detect high blood pressure, that of another person might take a much shorter time. However, studies have shown that specific breathing techniques could increase the sensitivity of baroreceptors, thus facilitating vagus nerve stimulation and reducing blood pressure.

Breathing Techniques that Can Stimulate the Vagus Nerve

The average human takes about 12 to 16 breaths per minute at rest. Deep and slow breathing reduces the number of breaths taken in a minute to induce relaxation via vagal stimulation.

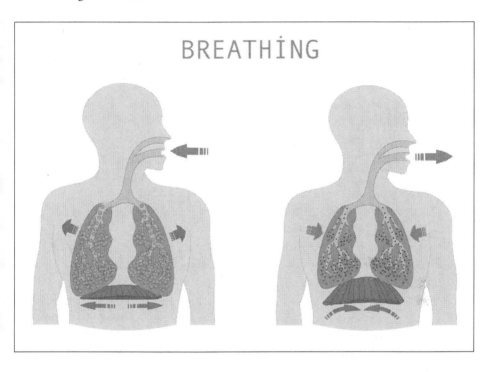

Immagine 7
Reiner hartmannpress

Here are a few breathing techniques that have been studied to have these effects:

1. **Ujjayi**: Ujjayi is a yogic slow breathing technique that allows an equal amount of time to breathe in and out. This technique can be performed at any rate as long as the same seconds are allocated for inhalation and

exhalation; however, the ideal rate is five seconds to breathe in and five seconds to breathe out. This involves a total of six breaths per minute.

2. **Box Breath**: Also known as square breath, this breathing technique involves an equal time of 4 seconds to inhale, hold, exhale and hold breath. This means that you are expected to breathe in for 4 sec, then hold your breath in for 4 sec, breathe out for another 4 sec and hold your breath for another 4 sec. A complete cycle takes 16 seconds, totalling almost four breaths in a minute and can be repeated for as long as you want.

3. **Alternate Nostril Breathing**: Also known as Nadi shodhana, alternate nostril breathing is another yogic breath control practice. It involves conscious inhalation through one nostril while the other is blocked, then exhaling through the previously blocked nostril while blocking the initial one. This cycle is then repeated between both nostrils in a regular pattern. This breathing pattern should be carried out 9 or 10 times before ending.

4. **4-7-8 Breathing**: This is a rhythmic breathing technique that involves emptying the lungs, breathing in quietly through the nose for a count of four seconds, holding the breath for 7 seconds, by exhaling through the mouth while making a 'whoosh' sound for 8 seconds and then repeating the cycle about 4 or 5 times. This breathing method is best carried out seated with your back straight.

5. **Lion's Breath**: Lion's breath is to be performed by sitting comfortably, preferably in a chair or on the floor, bracing your hands on your knees and spreading your fingers as possible. Then you must inhale through your nose, open your mouth, stick out your tongue, stretch it down towards your chin and exhale forcefully while making a 'ha' sound from your abdomen. You should breathe normally for a little while before doing the lion's breath again and repeat the cycle up to seven times.

6. **Pursed Lip Breathing**: This is yet another breathing technique, and it can either be carried out lying down or sitting with the back straight, and the shoulders relaxed. You are required to inhale through your nose for two seconds, making sure to fill your abdomen rather than your lungs, pucker your lips like you are about to give a kiss or blow air on a hot meal, exhale for four seconds and repeat the cycle.

7. **Resonant Breathing**: Also known as coherent breathing, this technique involves breathing in and out for a count of six seconds, thus totalling five full breaths in one minute. This pattern should be continued for about 10 minutes before stopping.

8. **Sitali Breath**: This breathing technique involves breathing in through the mouth, so before carrying it out, you want to ensure that you are in an environment with clean air. It would be best if you sat in a comfortable position, stuck out your tongue and folded it so that the outer edges are close together. If your language can't fold due to genetics, you can purse your lips, inhale and exhale through your nose. You should continue breathing like this for about 5 minutes.

9. **Diaphragmatic Breathing**: As the name implies, belly breathing involves breathing into the abdomen rather than the lungs. It can be performed sitting or lying. You must place one hand on your upper chest and the other on your belly below your ribcage. With your stomach relaxed, breathe in through your nose until you can feel your abdomen expand and exhale through slightly pursed lips while you can feel your belly fall towards your spine. Ensure that while you breathe, the hand on your chest remains still.

More tips on breathing slowly include:

- Assume a comfortable position with a good posture, either seating, standing, or laying
- Breath from your belly, expanding your abdomen and ribcage as you do so
- Inhale starting from the nose and exhale out the mouth
- Breath out for a longer time than you breathe in because relaxation is mainly triggered by slow exhalation

More tips on breathing slowly include:

- Inhale starting from the nose and exhale out the mouth
- Breath from your belly, expanding your abdomen and ribcage as you do so
- Breath out for a longer time than you breathe in because relaxation is mainly triggered by slow exhalation
- Other Health Benefits of Slow and Deep Breathing
- Intentional slow and deep breathing could help shift your focus from pain or stress. This is possible because the mind can only process one thing at a time, so if you concentrate on the rhythm and speed of your breathing, your mind is drawn away from the pain, reducing how much you can feel it.

- Conscious and slow breathing can help you breathe better if practised occasionally. It can help you have a better oxygen flow and strengthen your lung muscles while clearing the lungs to make room for more air.
- Deep breathing improves immunity by ensuring that the body gets more oxygen and promotes the exhalation of toxins and carbon dioxide, thus keeping the blood more oxygenated, cleaner and toxin-free
- Deep breathing can slow down the heart rate and balance cortisol levels in the body, thus providing relief from anxiety.
- Slow, deep, and long breaths can guarantee better sleep, especially in people with insomnia.
- Deep breathing increases a person's energy level by providing more oxygen to the blood.
- Deep breathing can help promote a better posture because most breathing exercises must be carried out in sitting, lying, or standing postures requiring a straight spine.
- Breathing exercises are a way of helping people who have lung conditions such as COPD and asthma to improve hyperventilation symptoms, lung function, and general lung efficiency.

Disadvantages of Slow and Deep Breathing

- It can cause chest pain in some people.
- It can present breathing difficulties in people with asthma, COPD, emphysema and bronchitis.
- It can easily be confused with big breathing

Cautions

Taking deep, slow, and conscious breaths differs from taking big breaths. Big breaths involve taking way more breath than needed, which can lead to over-breathing and mess with the cells' oxygen-carbon dioxide balance. It can also cause you to release too much carbon dioxide, thus impeding blood flow to the brain. Over-breathing or hyperventilation can also lead to:

- Lightheadedness
- Tiredness
- Hypoxia
- Tingling sensations
- Lower memory and concentration

6

COLD EXPOSURE

The Vagus nerve is the key to unlocking the body's natural ability to regulate stress, anxiety and depression.

COLD EXPOSURE

*S*tudies have shown that acute exposure to colds can stimulate the vagus nerve. This is because whenever the body is exposed and tries to adapt to cold temperatures, there is usually a decline in the sympathetic (flight or fight) system, which leads to an automatic increase in the parasympathetic (rest and digest) system. Since the vagus nerve is the main nerve of the parasympathetic system, this increase in the system's activity leads to its immediate stimulation.

Exposure to cold has also been shown to activate the cholinergic neurons, which are intrinsically found in the cerebral cortex, striatum, hippocampus, nucleus accumbens, and a few other areas. Cholinergic neurons make use of the neurotransmitter acetylcholine to send messages. Thus, increasing their activity could promote cortical activation during sleep and fine-tuning general brain function.

How To Make Use of Cold to Stimulate the Vagus Nerve

There are different ways through which you could expose yourself to cold temperatures. They include:

- **Coldwater immersion**: This method involves dunking a part of the body -mainly the face- or the whole body in ice-cold water. Full-body immersion in icy water is a practice that athletes usually carry out because it promotes relaxation. In the Scandinavian and Nordic regions, it is common to see people winter bathing, which involves swimming or dipping in frozen lakes or unheated pools.

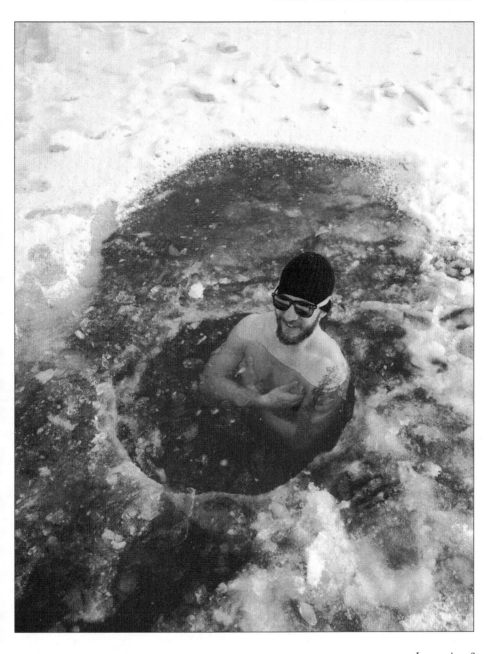

Immagine 8
Reiner hartmannpress

If you would instead not immerse your entire body in cold water, a simple

45

immersion of your face could also do the trick. You could also place an ice pack on your face or neck. These could be great ways for starters to ease themselves into the habit, and before long, you might find yourself ready to have your first full-body cold water immersion.

- Taking cold showers: A cold shower differs from a cold water immersion because it usually involves warmer waters and does not expose the entire body to cold. This implies that it might not be as effective as a complete immersion but could be more effective than a face immersion.

Getting used to a cold shower will likely take a while, but you can start by ending your regular batteries with about 30-60 seconds of cold water. With time, you could build your way up to more extended periods.

- Going out dressed in minimal clothing during cold weather. While this method does not involve direct skin contact with the cold like the two methods mentioned above, it is still very effective in stimulating the vagus nerve.

Other Health Benefits of Exposure to Cold

- Coldwater immersion or showers could increase the number of white blood cells in the body, thereby boosting the immune system and strengthening the body against illnesses such as the common cold.
- Exposing the body to cold could stimulate the release of hormones that trigger positive and pleasurable feelings, thus improving a person's mood and general mental state.
- Cold dips or showers help with weight loss by burning specific fat cells to generate heat.
- Exposure to cold triggers the release of cortisol, noradrenaline, and endorphins which can help with stress management, thus allowing a person to relax faster after moments of stress.
- Coldwater immersion can help improve blood circulation. To prevent body core temperature from dropping and ensure that the body extremities, such as fingers and toes, are kept warm, the heart pumps blood faster and harder around the body.

Disadvantages of Exposure to Cold
The use of cold to stimulate the vagus nerve has no known side effects or

consequences as long as it is carried out correctly. However, to promote the vagus nerve, you are advised not to expose yourself to chronic colds for extended periods, which could lead to specific respiratory and cardiovascular problems. These include:

- Shortness of breath
- Increase mucus secretion
- Cough Wheezing
- Chest pain
- Numbness
- Tickling sensation and change of colour in toes and fingers
- Stiffness
- Low body temperature
- Hypothermia

Cautions

The following persons are not advised to take cold showers or immerse themselves in cold water:

- People who are already complicated, as this could increase the time it takes to warm up and expose them to cold-related health problems
- People who are sick or under the weather because having to deal with the cold might be too much for their immune system to handle
- People who have heart diseases or are at a high risk of heart diseases because sudden exposure to cold could increase blood pressure and heart rate

7

SINGING, HUMMING, AND CHANTING

The Vagus nerve is the key to unlocking the body's natural ability to heal itself.

SINGING, HUMMING, AND CHANTING

he vagus nerve runs from the head down to the abdomen, encountering many organs on its way. In the neck and the throat, such organs that it faces and connects to are the vocal cords, the muscles at the back of the throat, and the inner ear. Since the vagus nerve connects to the vocal lines or voice box (larynx), making loud and energetic singing, humming, and chanting sounds can stimulate the nerve and increase the vagal tone. According to studies, these activities can also increase our heart rate variability, connected with stress resilience, adaptation, relaxation, and a general increase in parasympathetic (rest and digest) activity.

In one study to see how music affected the heart rate variability of a person singing, the authors theorized that singing could be compared to a vagal pump that sends relaxing waves through the vagus nerve with every note sung. Additionally, loud, energetic singing or singing at the top of your lungs can work the muscles at the back of your throat, thus activating the vagus nerve in the process, as well as increasing the activity of the sympathetic system, the combination of which could put one in a flow state.

In 2011, the International Journal of Yoga conducted another fascinating study to compare the differences between ÓM' chanting, 'Sss' pronunciation, and a state of rest. The study aimed to determine which exercises worked better to stimulate the vagus nerve. By the end of the study, it was discovered that 'OM' chanting was more effective than the other forms. This is because the chanting gives off a vibration around the ears and throughout the body that is picked up by the auricular branch of the vagus nerve, thus facilitating stimulation.

How to Sing, Hum and Chant to Stimulate the Vagus Nerve

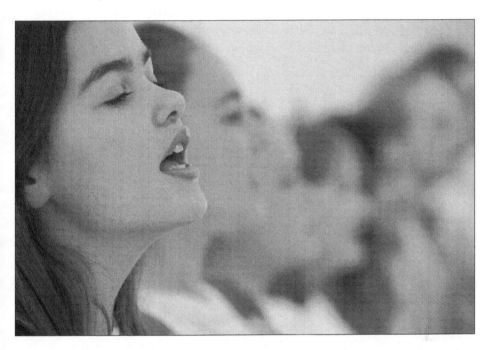

Immagine 9
Reiner hartmannpress

Only some were born with the musical ability to sing wonderfully or at very high pitches, and that's alright. Thankfully, you do not have to be a star in singing, humming, or chanting before you can activate your vagus nerve using these techniques. Here are a few ways through which you could carry out the exercises:

- **'OM' Chanting**: This involves chanting the word 'OM' long enough for effect. To chant this word, begin by chanting the vowel 'O' for a count of 5 seconds, then gradually begin chanting the consonant 'M' for 10 seconds. After a round of chanting, you can do some deep breathing before repeating the chant. Continue the cycle for about 10 minutes and conclude with some deep breathing.

- **Humming**: The main difference between singing and humming is that when you buzz, your mouth does not move, unlike during singing. Humming could either be done through the nose or the mouth. To perform the former, you can start by vocalizing a musical note or pitch while keeping your lips slightly parted, and your jaw, throat, and diaphragm relaxed. As you continue voicing the message, gradually bring your lips together until they are sealed, and no sounds can escape. The sound is then redirected to exit through your nose, thus creating a 'humming' noise.

To perform mouth humming, begin by humming, usually with your mouth closed and a relaxed jaw. Then slowly start to expand your throat as if you are trying to hit a shallow note. Do this until you feel your larynx begin to sink. Then with your lips tightly sealed, push from your diaphragm until you feel the vibrations fill up your cheeks. If you do it right, the lower part of your face and lips will tingle.

Sing: This is a straightforward and fun exercise. You can do this yourself, with your friends or kids, or in a choir. Also, you can sing along while playing a song, sing out a familiar tune, or be creative and sing out any sounds you like. However, how you choose to do it, ensure it is loud and energetic enough to engage your throat muscles and diaphragm.

Other Health Benefits of Singing, Humming, and Chanting

Asides from increasing parasympathetic (rest and digest) system activity and stimulating the vagus nerve, singing, humming, and chanting may offer the following health benefits:

- Some studies have shown that singing can reduce cortisol -the stress hormone- in individual saliva, thereby reducing the person's stress levels. However, cortisol only reduces when you sing in an environment that does not make you anxious or nervous, such as at a party, a gathering, or with friends.
- Signing can cause your body to release endorphins, a hormone that promotes positive feelings and can even increase a person's pain threshold.
- Singing regularly may positively affect how you breathe, and research carried out in 2008 shows that singing can be a potential treatment for snoring.

- Research has shown that chanting can reduce intrusive thoughts and mind wandering, making it easier for people to relax undisturbed and promote deep and restorative sleep.
- 'OM' chanting has been studied to improve mood, attention, and feelings of altruism or selflessness, thus making you a kinder, more affectionate version of yourself.
- Singing mostly involves the controlled use of throat muscles and some deep breathing, so it is beneficial for certain respiratory conditions, such as COPD and asthma, and other health conditions, including cystic fibrosis, cancer, quadriplegia, and multiple sclerosis.
- Singing and chanting in a group helps develop a sense of brotherliness and belonging, making people connect more easily.
- Humming can increase the amount of nitric acid produced by the nasal cells, a molecule responsible for increasing blood circulation and distributing oxygen to cells. Nitric acid could also affect sexual function, mood, and metabolic rate.
- Singing can enhance memory in people who have dementia or Alzheimer's. This is because not only can they remember lyrics and tunes, but some music could trigger the remembrance of specific life memories they had forgotten.
- Research has shown that singing can improve speech in people with speaking disabilities such as autism, Parkinson's disease, aphasia, and stuttering,

Disadvantages of Singing, Humming, and Chanting

- These activities could be distracting, primarily while working or studying.
- They could trigger bad or disturbing memories.
- Singing or humming could constitute noise pollution, especially when done loudly or in public spaces.

Caution

Too much of anything is terrible, and while singing is beautiful and uplifting, the same rule applies. Excessive singing, especially at a loud volume or high pitch, could cause a strain on the vocal cord, which, if care is not taken, could damage the voice box. Here are a few problems that might arise as a result of excessive singing:

- Vocal cord swelling: this can arise as a result of overuse or straining of your vocal cords. While this condition could vary from mild to severe, it usually does not cause permanent damage if treated by resting the vocal lines. Some symptoms of this condition include throat pain, speech difficulty, hoarseness, and persistent cough.
- A vocal cord nodule occurs when the repetitive and excessive use of the vocal cords leads to frequent swellings, and then the vocal lines begin to fold and get more challenging. As time passes, if this overuse of the vocal lines is not discontinued, it could lead to the nodules becoming more significant and more complex. Symptoms include neck pain, shooting pain through the ears, rough/scratchy voice, hoarseness, a lump in the throat, loss of voice, loss of vocal range, and breathiness.
- Vocal cord polyp: this can also be caused by overuse of the vocal cords, but unlike nodules that build up over time, polyps have been known to arise after just one occurrence of vocal abuse, for instance, a night of loud singing or shouting. They are usually red and vary in size. They share the same symptoms as nodules.

As a result, it is essential to exercise caution while singing to stimulate your vagus nerve. It would be best to avoid belting, yelling, screaming, shouting, straining to hit a note that is too high or too low, and anything that can be deemed too harsh. These precautions are essential to keep your vocal cords functioning at optimum levels.

8

MASSAGE THERAPY

The Vagus nerve is the body's built-in self-regulating system, helping to maintain physical and emotional balance.

A massage is an activity that involves the rubbing and kneading of the soft tissues and muscles of the body, manipulating them with gentle, or in some cases, intense pressure in a way that brings relief from pain and tension. Massage is one of the oldest therapy practised by the ancient Greeks, Egyptians, and Indians.

Massage therapy could be applied by making use of the hands, fingers, elbows, knees, forearms, feet, or a mechanical device not only has a good effect on the muscles and joints but could also be very beneficial to your bones heart, skin, mental health, breathing, and digestion - which brings us to the relationship of massage therapy to the vagus nerve.

Research has shown that massages on specific body parts can stimulate the vagus nerve; thus increasing vagal tone and activity, decreasing blood pressure and increasing heart rate variability. A vagus nerve massage does not work by massaging the vagus nerve itself but by rubbing the body parts closest to the nerve.

How to Use Massage Therapy to Stimulate the Vagus Nerve

Massage therapy can be applied to several body parts, ranging from the upper back to the lower back, arms, legs, butt, waist, neck, ears, eyes, and shoulders. The question is, 'Do massages of all these body parts automatically stimulate the vagus nerve?' Let's find out.

- **Neck massage**: The carotid arteries are located on either side of the neck, and their functions are to transport blood and oxygen to the head. Situated in the adventitia -the outermost layer- of the carotid artery is the carotid sinuses, which are baroreceptors that detect, respond and regulate systemic blood pressure.

Massaging the carotid sinus, which is located near the right side of the throat, helps stimulate the vagus nerve and may reduce seizures. However, we do not recommend that a carotid sinus massage be carried out at home or by an unprofessional. Additionally, it should not be performed on people with cardiovascular diseases. This is because, during the massage, the carotid artery could easily be blocked or restricted, leading to fainting and other health risks.

- **Pressure Massage**: This type of massage involves the application of sustained pressure to the inner layers of the muscles and connective tissues, using deep and slow strokes. The area of focus for this massage should be the gut which has even been shown to help babies increase weight due to vagus nerve stimulation.
- **Shoulder/neck/skull base massage**: The trapezius and sternocleidomastoid muscles can be found in the neck/shoulder area and the muscles below the base of the skull. The sternocleidomastoid muscles, located from the bottom of the head down to the sides of the neck, are responsible for tilting and rotating the head and keeping it aligned with the spine. In contrast, the trapezius muscles at the top of the shoulders are responsible for neck flexing and twisting shoulder movement, and head movement.

Research has shown that a massage of the base of the skull, shoulder, and neck, targeted at these muscles, can help stimulate the vagus nerve and increase heart rate variability.

- **Reflexology** involves gentle pressure on specific feet, ears, and hands points. This is an excellent option for people uncomfortable with being touched in the more intimate parts of their body, such as the back, waist, and thighs.

Aside from improving vagus activity and heart rate variability while reducing heart rate and blood pressure, it is also great for inducing relaxation, relieving pain, reducing fatigue, improving sleep, and much more. It can be carried out by rotating the ankles, stroking the soles gently, and stretching the toes back and forth.

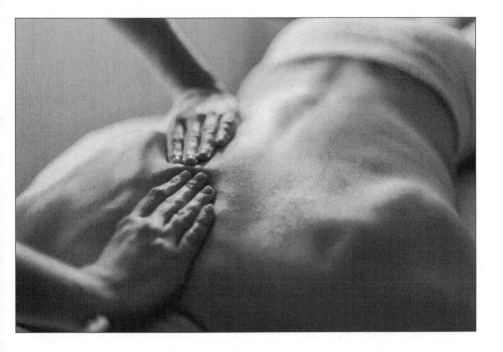

Immagine 10
Reiner hartmannpress

Other Health Benefits of Massage Therapy

- Massage therapy can help relieve stress-related problems, such as anxiety, panic attacks, and high blood pressure.
- Massages can help stimulate the lymphatic system.
- Massage therapy has also been proven to provide effective relief from pain, including back pain, arthritis (muscle and joint pain), and chronic pain.
- Massage therapy can be used in treating people with stroke
- Massages improve blood flow, thus increasing oxygen and nutrient distribution within the body's organs and tissues
- Massages can heighten your mental awareness
- Massages can eliminate toxins, harmful wastes, carbon dioxide, and excess water in the body.

- They can help prevent muscle or tissue damage, as well as help with rehab after an injury or accident.
- Massages can provide peace, calm, and euphoria and help you feel more comfortable in your body.

Disadvantages of Massage Therapy

While this procedure offers many health benefits, it could also have some side effects. However, these side effects are usually nothing to worry about because they are mild and should pass away in a few hours or days.

- Lingering pain as a result of unusual muscle movement and stimulation
- Muscle aches and soreness
- General fatigue and sleepiness
- Headaches or migraines
- Inflammation
- Skin irritation or redness
- Skin bruising

You should contact your doctor if these symptoms continue over a few days.

Caution

- Massage deals with manipulating soft tissues and muscles of the body, and if this is done with too much pressure, it could prove painful. This implies that rather than targeting and activating the vagus nerve, this massage could start the sympathetic (fight or flight) system, thus giving the opposite effect. As such, it is essential only to consult professionals for a massage.
- Avoid large meals or drinking alcohol before going for any massage treatment
- Inform your therapist if you think you might be or are pregnant
- Inform your therapist if you recently had surgery or any major injuries
- Inform your therapist if you have skin allergies

9

STRETCHING

The Vagus nerve is the key to unlocking the body's natural ability to cope with stress, anxiety and depression.

Stretching removes tension from muscles, joints, ligaments, and tendons by placing certain body parts in positions that will flex or lengthen them. Extension is also done to improve muscle elasticity and improve muscle tone. The effect of stretching is similar to that of massage, with the main difference being that during extension, there is no manipulation, kneading, or rubbing of the body.

A study has shown that stretching certain parts of the body can assist in stimulating the vagus nerve and help relieve anxiety and stress. Trying also has numerous health benefits that will be discussed later in this chapter. Now, let's take a quick look at the different types of stretching:

- **Static stretching**: This is a stretching that involves no movement at all. When doing this, you must get into your preferred stretch position and hold the place for a specific period, usually one minute. This stretching is generally done after strenuous physical activity such as a workout and is excellent for increasing blood flow and motion.
- **Dynamic stretching**: This type of stretching is carried out with movement. It involves making use of swinging or bouncing signals to carry out to activate the muscles. Unlike static stretching, dynamic

stretching does not precisely stretch out the strengths and is usually used as a warm-up for athletes or before a workout.

- **Passive stretching**: Passive stretching, as the name implies, is a form of extension that allows you to stay in one position without exactly doing anything. This stretching is usually carried out with the help of a partner, who does all the work for you by positioning a part of your body in a stretch position and holding it while you relax.
- **Proprioceptive Neuromuscular Facilitation (PNF) Stretching**: PNF stretching involves holding and releasing the stretched muscle to activate a maximum range of motion. It works by pulling a muscle to its limit, unleashing the power, and repeating the cycle until it is fully extended.

When concentrated in the right places, these stretches can activate the parasympathetic system and vagus nerve.

How to Use Stretching to Stimulate the Vagus Nerve

Any body part can be stretched, but that does not necessarily mean the vagus nerve is activated during the process. As a result, it is essential to know the exact body parts that are most effective for stretching.

- **Neck stretch**: The neck contains many muscles and nerve endings that make it stiff and tight and, simultaneously, very easy to activate. It would be best to be comfortable sitting in a chair or on the floor to carry out this exercise. Bring your right hand to the top of your head and gently lean your head towards your right shoulder. Your eyes should be tilted up to the Left when doing this.

It would be best if you held this position for a count of 30 seconds, keeping your head in the same place, after which you repeat the area with your left arm by leaning your head towards your left shoulder and holding for another 30 seconds.

- **Torso Stretch**: This stretch involves the same activity as the neck stretch above, only that this time, there is more action from the torso, precisely the rib cage. To carry out this stretch, get into a comfortable sitting position, either in a chair or on the floor. Place your right hand on the top of your head and your left hand reaching out to hold your right rib cage. To stretch, you lean your head towards your right shoulder and, using your left hand, pull your rib cage towards your left side, as though trying to form a 'C' shape with your spine.

Hold this position for 30 seconds and try not to strain too much. When done with your right side, you should move to your left side and repeat the same process with your left hand on your head and your right hand holding your left rib cage.

- **Ear Stretch**: The ear connects to some parts of the vagus nerve and can stimulate it. First, place a finger on the ridge of your ear canal in both ears and move in small circles. Please do this for a while, then switch to pull your ears away from your skull and move them in upward and downward strokes. Asides from stimulating the vagus nerve, this could also help relieve headaches.

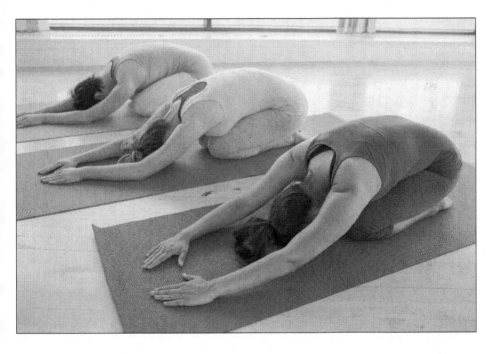

Immagine 11
Reiner hartmannpress

Other Health Benefits of Stretching

- Stretching provides relief from discomfort in the body caused by tension and stress build-up.
- Stretching can improve circulation by allowing more blood flow to muscles, thus reducing muscle soreness and shortening recovery time.

- Stretching can reduce the impact of ageing on the body and make you look younger than you are
- Stretching increases flexibility, which makes it easier to perform daily activities with ease
- Stretching can increase your range of motion.
- Stretching can be used as a warm-up for physical activities to improve your performance.
- Stretching some muscles in the body can help improve body posture and promote proper bone alignment.
- Stretching can help prevent and relieve pain
- Stretching is excellent for relieving stress and calming the mind

Disadvantages of Stretching

Like several other exercises, stretching can be dangerous and harmful, primarily when not appropriately performed.

Research has shown that stretching could cause a reduction in muscle power and force production capacity, thus leading to weakness in the muscle.

- Research has shown that stretching could increase the risk of injuries in athletes.
- Research has shown that when a stretched muscle is weakened, the brain might be triggered to weaken other muscles, even if they are not tested.
- Stretching can cause extended muscle problems lasting up to a week or more.
- Stretching can cause damage or tears in muscles and connective tissues
- Stretching can make muscles too loose, thus putting a strain on the joints and increasing the risks of injury

Cautions

Stretching might only sometimes be a safe practice, especially in the presence of certain factors. Here are a few safety tips to note:

- If you have an existing injury or a nagging injury, ensure that you speak to a professional to help you draw up exercises that are suitable for your needs, and make sure to perform only these recommended stretches
- Do not carry out stretches that require you to bounce unless they have been expressly recommended by a professional

- Stay within the point of comfort. You might feel tension while stretching, but you should never feel pain. If you are feeling pain, stop trying that particular muscle.
- Don't stretch cold muscles. Ensure to do a little warm-up to make the muscles more pliable.
- Do not hold your breath while stretching, which could increase muscle tension. Instead, take deep and slow breaths as you stretch.
- If it is not tight, do not stretch it. Rather than work on a muscle that is not tight, figure out the tight muscles in your body and increase their flexibility.
- Most importantly, please do just what is necessary.

1 0

YOGA

The Vagus nerve is the body's natural defense mechanism, helping us to recover from trauma and injury.

*Y*oga is a ubiquitous word in the world today. However, only a few people realize how well this exercise can help them achieve the desired well-being of body and mind. Many people think yoga is just about physical poses when it involves several self-disciplinary practices.

Yoga is a physical activity that involves body positioning accompanied by breathing exercises, meditation, and relaxation to exercise the mind and the body. Yoga also includes chanting, mantra, prayer, ritual, and selfless action.

Scientific research into yoga and its health benefits still needs to be completed. However, all evidence point to the fact that it provides support for overall physical and mental health, and a few studies have suggested that there might be a link between yoga and vagus nerve stimulation. Yoga also activates the parasympathetic (rest and digest) system by increasing blood flow and aiding digestion.

There are six main branches of yoga, all targeted at different aspects of living, and they include:

- **Hatha yoga**: This branch deals with physical and mental practices that prime the body and mind
- **Raja yoga**: This branch desks with meditation and strict observation to several self-disciplinary steps, also known as the eight limbs of yoga

- **Karma yoga**: This branch is a path of service that targets the creation of a future that is rid of negativity and selfishness
- **Bhakti yoga**: This branch is targeted at creating a positive way to channel emotions and increase acceptance and tolerance
- **Jnana yoga**: This branch of yoga deals with wisdom and the development of the intellect through study
- **Tantra yoga**: This branch links meditative and yogic practices together to promote feelings of self-love and acceptance

How to Use Yoga to Stimulate the Vagus Nerve

Yogic practices are available in abundance, and while every single one has its benefits, some specific ones can trigger the vagus nerve more effectively. Here are some yoga practices that you could try:

1. **Half smile**: Some part of the vagus nerve extends into the face muscles, and thus, these muscles can be worked on to increase vagal tone. Aside from its ability to improve a person's mental state and increase feelings of positivity, a smile, or in this case, a half-smile is effective in stimulating the vagus nerve. As you turn your lips in a smile, picture your jaws softening and releasing the tension in them, and imagine a feeling of relaxation spreading around your face, across your head, and down to your shoulders. This simple activity could increase your parasympathetic (rest and digest) system function.
2. **Open your heart posture**: This yoga posture is said to open the heart and throat, thus increasing circulation and vagal tone. To carry it out, assume a comfortable position, bring your hands to the top of your shoulders and gently exhale. As you do this, expand the front of your chest, spread your elbows wide and raise your chin. Hold this position for a while, and when you are exhaling, contract your elbows to the front of your chest and drop your chin. Repeat this cycle several times, and ensure to focus on the inhaling part of the breathing part.
3. **Release the tension in your eyes**: Have you ever wondered why you could notice if a person is stressed just by looking into their eyes? This is because the 12 extraocular muscles of the eye are directly connected to the vagus nerve. This implies that eye movement can stimulate the vagus nerve by improving the blood flow to the vertebral artery. Equally, relaxing the eye muscles can reduce heart rate and blood pressure by activating the functioning of the parasympathetic (rest and digest) system.

To relax the eyes, you should apply gentle pressure by placing your palms over the eyes or pressing down gently. You could also place an eye pillow over your eyes as you sleep or relax. Ensure you do not apply too much pressure to prevent loss of consciousness.

The vagus nerve can also be activated through eye movement. To do this, hold a pencil or any small object about five inches from your face, and focus your eyes on this object for anywhere between 20 and 30 seconds. Then, shift your eyes from the thing and stare into space for another 20 to 30 seconds. Repeat this cycle a few times, after which you can then relax your eyes.

- **Yoga Nidra**: This restorative yoga can slow down and calm the nervous system by assessing and restoring the parasympathetic nervous system. To perform this exercise, assume a comfortable position on the floor, with a yoga mat or blanket underneath you for comfort. Grow a consciousness of your breath and body in general. Create a space for whatever emotion you feel in that moment, including all the tension and heaviness. Remain still in this position for about 30 minutes. When you are done, you should feel the heaviness and pressure gone.
- **Release the belly posture**: The vagus nerve extends into the abdominal cavity and can thus be activated by some postures that affect the stomach muscles. To practice this exercise, get on the floor with your hands under your shoulders and your knees under your hips, like a table. The idea is to breathe in and out in this position. When you inhale, raise your head and hips while lowering your belly towards the floor and moving into a cow pose. Refer to the image below for reference. When you exhale, lower your head and hips and raise your spine into a cat pose. It would be best if you repeated this movement as many times as possible, making sure to find a time that suits you. This exercise is a massage for your spine and belly and can activate the vagus nerve if done correctly.

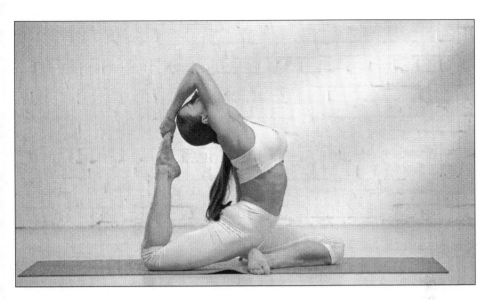

- **Easy seated twist**: Also known as Parvrtta Sukhasana, this exercise helps to move the spine, belly, chest, and throat. You can carry this out sitting in a chair or on the floor. Place your left hand on the outside of your right leg and your right hand behind you, thus assuming a twist position. When you inhale, straighten your spine, and when you exhale, increase your twist, inclining your spine towards the right. While doing this, you can tilt your chin towards the right and look over your shoulder.

Take several breaths in this position before returning to the initial work and repeating the same breathing pattern on your left side. Once done, return to the centre and note your body's general feeling.

Other Health Benefits of Yoga

There is no doubt about the fact that yoga offers several benefits to people who practice it, including an improvement in mental health, emotional health, and physical health.

- Some studies have shown that yoga can increase flexibility, even in older adults over 65. This is because it offers a wide range of postures and exercises that vary in intensity from mild to high, thus allowing people to ease their muscles into flexibility slowly.

- Yoga, physical and mental practices, such as meditation, chanting, sound baths, and breathwork, have been proven to relieve stress.
- Studies support that yoga is an effective treatment of mental health issues, including major depressive disorder (MDD)
- Yoga may reduce inflammation caused by chronic diseases such as arthritis, diabetes, heart disease, and Crohn's disease.
- Yoga is an effective strength-building practice.
- Other studies suggest that yoga may be an effective treatment for anxiety disorders.
- Some studies show that there might be a link between yoga and a boost to the immune system.
- Yoga can improve balance, even in older adults, thus reducing the risks of falls.
- Yogic breath work can improve the functioning of the cardiovascular system.
- Yoga can help treat insomnia, thus helping people fall asleep quicker, sleep more profoundly, and stay asleep longer.
- Yoga may improve a person's perception of themselves, thus improving self-esteem, especially in adolescents and teenagers.
- Yoga can increase the spine's mobility, reduce muscle tightness and improve bone alignment, thus improving posture.
- Yoga can increase bone density and improve general bone health

Disadvantages of Yoga

Some poses in yoga might not be as safe as we like to think they are. If it is overdone, yoga can result in the following:

- Repetitive strain injuries
- Nerve damage
- Foot weakness
- Degenerative arthritis of the cervical spine
- Increased risks of spinal compression and fractures
- Overstretching of nerve tissue
- Hip injuries and damage
- Increased risk for stroke

Cautions

Yoga is generally considered to be safe, especially when practised with a well-trained instructor. However, the following people should consider some risk factors before beginning yoga:

- Pregnant people should consult with a professional to determine which exercises are safe before taking up yoga
- People with an ongoing medical condition, such as glaucoma or bone loss, should consult with their healthcare provider before practising yoga
- If you are a beginner, avoid practising advanced techniques and challenging poses

GARGLING

*G*argling is an act of bubbling liquid in the mouth by breathing through it with a gurgling sound. It is a home remedy for certain conditions, including sore throat, mouth sores, canker sores, allergic reactions, respiratory infections, and other conditions that affect the throat and mouth.

Although no proper research has been carried out into the effect of gargling on the vagus nerve, it is believed by many experts that gargling may help in activating the vagus nerve. This is because gargling contracts the muscles at the back of the throat, thus starting the vagus nerve and stimulating the gastrointestinal tract. Also, the physical repercussion of the vocal cords can activate the vagus nerve, according to D'Elia Assenza. Since gargling causes this reverberation, then it can be employed to stimulate the vagus nerve.

How To Use Gargling to Stimulate the Vagus Nerve

To gargle, pour yourself a cup of water, tilt your head back, and pour some of the water - a quantity you are comfortable with- into your mouth without drinking it. Keep your epiglottis closed during this period to prevent drinking the water. Gargle the water vigorously for between 20 and 30 seconds before swallowing the water.

Pour more water from the cup into your mouth and repeat the process for 20 or 30 seconds. Repeat this cycle until the cup is empty. If you do it right, you might begin tearing up. If you do not tear up, we encourage you to keep gargling until you can feel yourself start to tear up slightly.

It would be best to Gargled about four or five times daily and for long periods to ensure its effectiveness in stimulating your vagus nerve.

Other Health Benefits of Gargling

Saltwater gargles are very effective in the treatment of certain oral conditions. It is a simple home remedy made out of water and salt. Studies show that salt can be used to draw moisture out of the tissues and, at the same time, prevent harmful pathogens from getting in.

- Saltwater gargling can be effective in the treatment of sore throats. They provide relief from discomfort caused by inflammation and can keep the mouth clean, and prevent infections.
- Saltwater gargling can help reduce the severity of sinus and respiratory infections caused by viruses or bacteria. These infections include cold, strep throat, flu, and mononucleosis.
- Saltwater neutralizes the acids in the mouth that cause the multiplication of bacteria.
- Gargling can improve gum and dental health and prevent gingivitis, periodontitis, and cavities.
- Salt Water gargling can effectively treat stomach ulcers, also known as canker sores.

Disadvantages of Gargling

Gargling is generally considered to be safe for children and adults. There are no clear dangers from carrying out this activity.

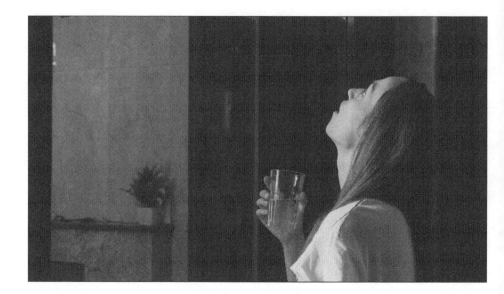

Immagine 13
Reiner hartmannpress

Cautions

Here are some precautions that might help make gargling more effective and safer:

- Do not use hot water when gargling. Warm water is preferable to prevent blisters in the mouth or throat
- Only clean water in a clean cup should be used for gargling. Preferably, set a cup aside for this purpose
- Always tilt your head backwards when gargling to ensure that the throat is touched properly
- If you are gargling with anything other than plain water, such as mouthwash or saltwater, try to ensure the liquid does not enter the throat. Saltwater could lead to dehydration, and mouthwashes are dangerous to swallow in large quantities.
- Do not let a child less than six years old gargle.
- Only people who know how to gargle should gargle. If you cannot gargle or if you find it difficult, do not force it.

ASMR (AUTONOMOUS SENSORY MERIDIAN RESPONSE)

The Vagus nerve is the body's secret weapon in the fight against anxiety and depression.

*a*utonomous Sensory Meridian Response (ASMR) is a term that describes a tingling and calming sensation that starts at the top of the head and travels down the spine and limbs. In recent years, many people have begun to seek out videos on social media that activate this response because of how calming and thrilling they can be. There are, in fact, over 10 million ASMR-related videos on the internet. Despite the overwhelming attention that it is receiving, there have been a few scientific studies on the subject.

However, anecdotally, much evidence suggests that ASMR can be triggered in people through audio and visual means. Not everyone experiences ASMR, however, so while one person might get moved from hearing certain sounds or sights, others might not. ASMR can be triggered by sounds and companies such as tapping of fingers, light touches, soft sounds, popping, delicate hand movements, accentuated sounds, rustling noises, sounds of water, crinkling, swishing, blowing, scratching, tearing, mixing, and squashing.

In a study conducted on 1,000 people who watched both ASMR-related videos and videos with no ASMR content, the participants who said they were mainly triggered also recorded the highest levels of calm feelings. The same research also showed that people who experienced ASMR sensations had a lower heart rate than others who did not frequently experience these sensations. These people also reported feeling less stressed, less harmful, and more positive.

Reducing heart rate and stress levels is synonymous with increased parasympathetic (rest and digest) function. Since the vagus nerve is the main nerve of this system, then it goes without saying that ASMR could stimulate the vagus nerve.

How to Use Autonomous Sensory Meridian Response to Stimulate the Vagus Nerve

ASMR-triggering contents are all over the internet space. If you have never heard of or watched one, go on to Youtube and search 'ASMR'. You should note that not everyone feels this sensation, and different sounds trigger it in other people. It might take you a while to find out what sounds do it for you, and once you do, you can be on your way to stimulating your vagus nerve by just listening and watching.

As mentioned above, two significant stimuli trigger ASMR sensations, and they are visual and auditory stimuli. The sounds below shall be divided based on these categories.

Auditory Triggers

The following are sounds that have been reported to help people achieve a state of calm and trigger an auto-sensory meridian response:

- **Whispering**: Whispering is speaking in hushed tones and an unvoiced manner. While you might be able to make out the words in some cases, other times, you can't. Certain people find that hearing whispering incredibly close to their ears triggers a sensation in their bodies.
- **Page turning**: This involves a papery sound that can be gotten from turning the pages of a book, glossy magazine, newspaper, or other papery objects. These sounds are usually enhanced and made more prominent and bolder to create a sensation in people listening.
- **Writing**: Listening to a pencil or pen scratch against the surface of a paper might be comforting to some people and assist them in feeling ASMR sensations.
- **Crisp sounds**: These sounds like crinkly, wrinkly, or cracking sounds that you might get from crumpling a sheet of paper, a roll of foil or dry leaves, and a noisy rocking chair. Hearing these sounds close up may elicit a tinkling or warm sensation in your body.
- **Tapping**: A steady-rhythmic tapping sound echoing from fingernails or fingertips tapping against a hard surface like a tabletop, glass bottle, keyboard, or a softer surface like a candle or carton could also evoke ASMR sensations.

- **Scratching**: The sound made from rubbing the nails against dry surfaces, such as a book cover, a wicker basket, a wooden door, or a wall, has also been calming and relaxing.
- **Munching and swirling**: Hearing sounds from food chewing, drinking, crunching, gnawing, and nail clipping or liquids mixing in the mouth can also trigger these feelings in people.

Visual Triggers
The following are sights that have been reported to help people achieve a state of calm and trigger an auto-sensory meridian response:

- **Small, slow movements**: Small movements like trailing a fingernail or fingertip against bare skin, writing, making slow and calculated hand gestures, or rocking slowly in a chair may trigger sensations in certain people.
- **Brush strokes**: A small makeup brush stroking against a powder palette or a paintbrush moving silently across paper can also evoke relaxing and calming feelings in some people.
- **Hair brushing**: Watching a comb or hair brush run slowly through hair or brushing the fur of a pet, such as a dog or a cat, can elicit a sense of calm and comfort in many people. In the same way, having your hair combed, stroked, or played with can make a person feel relaxed or sleepy.
- **Stroking a pet**: Cuddling a pet closely and slowly running fingers through its fur can help some people feel calm and comforted, especially if this is combined with purring sounds from the pet and the human.
- **Stretching and mixing wax or slime**: Stretching out and mixing mud or spreading wax on the part of the skin can make some people feel ASMR sensations.

13

LAUGHTER

Meditation and deep breathing activate the Vagus nerve, promoting a sense of calm and relaxation.

ou know the saying, "Laughter is the best medicine." That's what we've always been told, but did you know it's true, especially concerning the vagus nerve? While it may not be top on our list of exercises, it is one very effective way to stimulate the vagus nerve. Laughter also offers many health benefits, including physical and emotional changes in the body.

Laughing is an excellent way to keep your mind and body healthy. It can also be a great form of stress relief. A study from the University of Maryland found that laughing can stimulate the vagus nerve. When you laugh, your diaphragm contracts and pushes air out of your lungs. This causes a rush of air through your nasal passages and throat, stimulating the nerves that run along these pathways— particularly those in your larynx and sinuses. This stimulation triggers a signal sent to your brain stem, activating the vagus nerve.

The vagus nerve then sends signals to your organs, telling them to relax and slow down their activity levels. This helps regulate blood pressure and heart rate and reduces stress on the digestive system. Laughter has also been shown to increase heart rate variability, directly connected to vagus nerve functioning.

How to Stimulate the Vagus Nerve Using Laughter

There is no exact way of teaching someone how to laugh. It is an automated reaction that comes from within a person. While some people may find laughing easy, it could be harder for others. However, specific triggers can make you laugh more efficiently and genuinely. Let's take a look at those:

- **Surprise**: The element of surprise is one method that has been proven to evoke laughter in people. Imagine that you have not seen a loved one in a while, and out of the blue, they show up on your doorstep one Sunday afternoon. As you throw yourself into their arms, you will likely laugh.

Another instance is a funny plot twist you didn't see in your favourite TV series. The feelings of surprise come alongside laughter and cheers.

- **Embarrassment**: Nobody likes to get embarrassed; honestly, a burst of embarrassed laughter is not exactly the best form of laughter. But it is laughter all the same, and it could quickly transform into something more profound, especially if you are in the company of friends. This is also great because it would make you laugh and make the people around you laugh, even if it's just for a bit.
- **Watch something funny**: This is one of the purest ways of getting yourself to laugh. The internet is crawling with many funny videos and clips, all targeted at making people laugh and feel good. Funny videos range from sitcoms to stand-up comedies, short skits, and humorous scenes from movies. Asides from watching, you could also listen to funny audio or read comics.
- **Spend time with loved ones**: One of the best and most trusted ways to laugh is to spend time with people who make you happy. This includes friends, family, and lovers. Taking time out of your busy life to meet with friends or have dinner with your family might help you loosen up, play, laugh, and ultimately feel better.

When together with your loved ones, play games that can elicit a feeling of togetherness and help you bond and laugh. Such games include board games, charades, hide and seek, dress-up, and more.

- **Make memories**: Have you ever suddenly remembered something funny that you saw, heard, or experienced in the past and suddenly burst out laughing? Well, that was simply because you made the memory in the first place. Engage in activities that will leave a dent of fun in your memory. Travel, visit classes, engage in sports, hit the club, or meet new people.

Other Health Benefits of Laughing

Laughing is an excellent way to get your daily dose of exercise. You are having a good time this time rather than straining and sweating. Asides from stimulating the vagus nerve, here are some health benefits of laughing:

- Scientific research shows that laughing can increase the endorphins in your body, hormones that make you feel good. These hormones can reduce pain and depression symptoms, enhance mood, and decrease stress.
- Laughing may help you live longer by reducing blood pressure and heart rate and strengthening the heart muscles, thus lessening the risks of cardiovascular occurrences.
- Studies have shown that laughing is effective in improving lung function and boosting immune system activity (American Heart Association)
- Laughing significantly increases the flow of oxygen-rich blood to the brain, which can help you think clearly and quickly and increases your attention span and memory.
- Laughing is a great way to relax and relieve stress

Dangers of Laughing

Laughing in itself is not the problem. The problem is laughing too hard. Laughing too hard can be very dangerous, like the Greek philosopher Chrysippus, who died shortly after laughing at his joke. Although there is no proof to back it up, many people believe he died from laughing too hard.

Laughing by itself does not kill. However, it can trigger certain conditions that could be life-threatening. They include:

- **Broken brain aneurysm**: A brain aneurysm is a blood vessel swelling in the brain. Its cause is unknown and can go undiagnosed for a long time. If you have a brain aneurysm, laughing too hard may rupture it, thus leading to bleeding in the brain, brain damage, and increased pressure in the skull cavity. Symptoms include confusion, double vision, vomiting, severe headache, seizures, and sensitivity to light.
- **Asthma attack**: Asthma attacks can be provided by various factors, including allergies, physical exercises, lousy weather, and, yes, laughing. Laughing too hard could cause a severe asthma attack, making it difficult to breathe, and if medical help is not provided, this attack could become fatal.

- **Suffocation**: Extended laughter can prevent air from getting into the lungs, thus depriving the body of oxygen and could lead to death.
- **Syncope** is referring to a temporary loss of consciousness because of insufficient blood flow to the brain. It can be caused by dehydration, exhaustion, low blood pressure, or a low heart rate. Aside from these reasons, however, it can also be caused by hard laughing. While this may not result in a cardiac arrest, it could lead to severe injuries from you falling.
- **Gelastic seizures**: These are seizures associated with uncontrollable laughter either while sleeping or awake. In this case, the victim cannot stop laughing, and these seizures could be life-threatening.

So remember, it is perfectly okay to laugh. It is okay to laugh out loud, also. Death by laughter is not a common occurrence and can be avoided. If you develop weird symptoms after a laughing fit, report them to your healthcare provider to prevent complications.

1 4

ACUPUNCTURE

The Vagus nerve is the body's connection to the mind-body connection, helping us to understand and regulate our emotions.

*a*cupuncture is a very old Chinese practice that uses fragile needles to stimulate the body's energy flow. It effectively treats various conditions, from depression and anxiety to chronic pain and even cancer.

Acupuncture can help you to relax, reduce stress and anxiety, and feel more energized. It works by stimulating the energy flow (Qi) through your body's meridians, which are pathways through which Qi flows. The goal is to balance Yin and Yang—the opposing yet complementary forces in the body that regulate all biological processes—and the Five Elements: Wood, Fire, Earth, Metal, and Water.

One of the most common questions about acupuncture is how it works: how does sticking needles into your skin affect your body?

The answer lies in the vagus nerve, which connects to our heart, lungs, stomach, liver, gallbladder, pancreas, and intestines. It also connects to our eyes and ears, so acupuncture can treat headaches or hearing loss.

Acupuncture stimulates this nerve by inserting needles into specific points on your skin, known as acupoints. The needle insertion may cause some discomfort initially but isn't painful after a few minutes. These pain-sensing neurons (called nociceptors) are activated by activating TRPV1 receptors on these neurons.

These receptors are activated by capsaicin (also produced by chilli peppers). When activated this way, they cause sodium channels to open and potassium media to close—leading to depolarization of the cell membrane and calcium ions influx into the cell. This influx triggers an electrical signal down the axon of these neurons and eventually reaches your brain stem, where it stimulates the vagus nerve.

How to Use Acupuncture to Stimulate the Vagus Nerve

Acupuncture is a special treatment that a professional should carry out. It is not a do-it-yourself (DIY) procedure and should not be treated as such. Your acupuncturist will know how to insert the needles to aid the vagus nerve activation. You do not require any special preparations when going for an acupuncture treatment.

However, because the success or failure of this procedure lies solely in the hands of your acupuncturist, it is crucial to consider selecting one for yourself. Here are several things you should consider:

- The acupuncturist's credentials and training. Typically, acupuncture practitioners are required to pass an exam led by the National Certification Commission for Acupuncture and Oriental Medicine.
- Ask the acupuncturist questions about the treatment, including its cost, what it entails and how it will help your condition.
- Get recommendations from people you trust and your doctor.

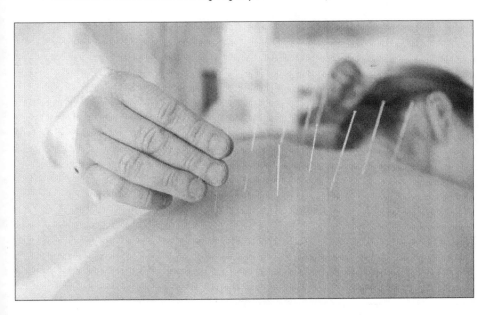

Immagine 14

Other Health Benefits of Acupuncture

- Acupuncture is a practice that has been around for thousands of years, but it's only recently that we've begun to understand how it works. It offers tons of benefits to the human body, including the following:
- Acupuncture stimulates the release of neurotransmitters like serotonin and endorphins - which are responsible for regulating moods like anxiety and depression as well as oxytocin -which helps us feel connected with others (this might be why many people say that getting acupuncture reminds them of their moms!)
- Acupuncture can help you feel more relaxed by stimulating blood flow through meridians and increasing oxygen levels in the body. This can help you feel less stressed when you're experiencing pain or other symptoms of stress, such as headaches or insomnia.
- Acupuncture may increase your energy reserve and make you feel better equipped to handle your usual activities.
- Acupuncture can provide relief for people suffering from insomnia
- Acupuncture may strengthen the immune system and help build resistance to diseases
- Acupuncture could relieve pain such as headaches, back pain, labour pain, menstrual cramps, neck pain, and dental pain

Dangers of Acupuncture

Acupuncture is considered a safe practice. However, it could come with its dangers and side effects. Possible risks of acupuncture include:

- Soreness, bruising, or bleeding at the sites where the needles are inserted
- The use of non-sterile needles can cause infections
- Although very rare, a hand could break inside the body and rupture an internal organ

Caution

If you have the following conditions, it is advisable to inform your acupuncturist about it before going ahead with the process:

- If you are pregnant, this is because some acupuncture spots can induce labour and, if triggered during your treatment, could lead to premature delivery.
- If you have bleeding disorders, although acupuncture does not exactly result in bleeding, there is a higher chance that you would bleed from the insertion points if you have a bleeding disorder or are on blood thinners.
- If you have a pacemaker, sometimes, an acupuncturist may apply slight electrical charges to the inserted needles, which could disrupt the pacemaker's rhythm.

15

OTHER WAYS TO IMPROVE YOUR VAGAL TONE

The Vagus nerve is the body's built-in self-regulating system, helping to maintain balance in the face of stress and adversity.

From all that has been said, there is no doubt that the vagus nerve is essential to an individual's everyday life; hence, there is a need to ensure the seamless functionality of the vagus nerve. This chapter emphasizes other ways of enhancing vagal tone outside the methods discussed earlier. These methods may be for medical purposes or to strengthen and improve your vagal tone.

Probiotics and prebiotics

With the understanding of the relationship between the vagus nerve and gut microflora, it is no surprise that a healthy microbiota system in the gut is beneficial to vagus nerve health and recovery. It has been established that humans and microorganisms work in mutualism. They need us to release the products they consume, and we need them for various bodily and environmental functions. Probiotics and prebiotics help to stimulate the growth of microflora in the body, especially gut microbiota, and these organisms, in turn, secrete chemical substances. These chemical substances increase the stimulation of the vagus nerve via the gut-brain axis, thus, improving vagal tone.

In addition to boosting vagal tone, probiotics and prebiotics are believed to increase gut barrier and resistance to keep out harmful substances, viruses, and bacteria. This, in turn, helps to reduce inflammation and may potentially reduce cancer risk. Also, by boosting the growth and activities of gut microorganisms, probiotics and prebiotics assist in digestion and absorption, especially digestion of vitamin K and fatty acids.

Probiotics

Probiotics are living microorganisms consumed in adequate but healthy amounts to provide health benefits for the host. Some of these beneficial microorganisms consumed include:

- Lactobacillus bulgaricus
- Leuconostoc mesenteroides
- Lactobacillus plantarum
- Pediococcus pentosaceus
- Lactobacillus brevis
- Leuconostoc citreum
- Leuconostoc argentinum
- Lactobacillus para plantarum
- Lactobacillus coryniformis
- Weissella app
- Lactobacillus acidophilus
- Saccharomyces boulardii
- Bifidobacterium bifidum
- Streptococcus thermophilus
- Lactobacillus helveticus
- Lactobacillus kefiranofaciens
- Lactococcus lactis.

Food and drinks that contain probiotics include:

- Kimchi
- Buttermilk
- Kombucha
- Kefir
- Sauerkraut
- Pickles
- Miso
- Tempeh
- Sourdough bread
- Cheese.

Although the consumption of probiotics is relatively safe with no adverse effects, specific individuals may be at risk of developing unfavourable effects. Such individuals include those with:

- Immunodeficiency disorders like chronic granulomatous disease
- Short bowel syndrome
- Central venous catheters
- Cardiac valve disease
- Individuals who just had surgery
- Premature infants.

Prebiotics

Prebiotics is generally a term used to describe foods that promote microbial growth, especially in the gut. Dietary prebiotics is usually indigestible fibre compounds that remain undigested as they move through the gastrointestinal tract- from the mouth and stomach to the intestines. They can help stimulate the growth and activity of these beneficial bacteria in the colon by acting as substrates or fertilizers. Hence, these particular compounds and substances in these foods serve as a source for the growth and activity of valuable microorganisms such as bacteria and fungi.

Some of these beneficial microorganisms include Bifidobacteria and Lacto-bacillus. With improvement in scientific technology over the years, the modern prebiotic targets have increased to include a broader range of microbes such as Roseburia spp., Eubacterium app., Akkermansia spp., Christensenella spp, Propionibacterium spp. and Faecalibacterium spp.

Before food or any substance qualifies as prebiotics, it must meet the following criteria:

- It must be non-digestible and resistant to enzymatic activities by stomach acid and enzymes in the human gastrointestinal tract
- Microorganisms on or in the body can ferment it
- It must be able to stimulate the growth and activity of beneficial bacteria in the body

Foods that are prebiotics-rich include:

- Garlic
- Chicory
- Onions

- Asparagus
- Konjac root
- Bananas
- Barley
- Leeks
- Dandelion Greens
- Wheat Bran
- Ginger
- Apples
- Flaxseed.

Vagus Nerve Stimulation Devices

In severe cases, specific individuals may present to a hospital with a shallow vagal tone and stimulation or other nervous system abnormalities like epilepsy, which would mainly require medical intervention. Vagus nerve stimulation is a significant medical intervention for such individuals, especially if they are not responding to medication.

Vagus nerve stimulation entails implanting an artificial device that stimulates the vagus nerve by sending mild electrical impulses through the nerve to the brain. During the procedure, a cut is made on the skin of the upper left chest, and the device's generator is embedded in a little sac under the collarbone. A second incision is made in the neck so the surgeon can access the vagus nerve.

The surgeon then attaches the leads around the left branch of the vagus nerve and links the electrodes to the generator. Once the device is adequately implanted and tested and the rate of electrical impulse generated is set, the generator sends electric impulses to the vagus nerve at regular intervals. In vagus nerve stimulation, the left vagus nerve is stimulated instead of the right because the right nerve plays a vital role in regulating cardiac function. If encouraged, it could result in adverse cardiac consequences.

However, it is essential to know that vagus nerve stimulation may only be ideal for some. The Vagus nerve is contraindicated in the following conditions:

- Pregnancy
- Respiratory and lung disorders include asthma, chronic obstructive pulmonary disease, etc.
- Active peptic ulcer disease
- Diabetes mellitus, particularly insulin-dependent
- Presence of only one vagus nerve or previous surgery to remove part of the vagus nerve

85

- Disorders that influence the normal functioning of the autonomic nervous system.
- The individual is currently receiving other forms of brain stimulation or therapy.
- Abnormal cardiac conditions like arrhythmias
- History of abnormal psychological disorders such as schizophrenia, schizoaffective disorder, delusional disorders, or rapid cycling bipolar disorder.

Maintaining a Healthy Lifestyle
The benefits of developing healthy habits should be balanced as this improves vagal tone and enhances an individual's quality of life and overall health.

Defecate Regularly
Bowel movement and defecation are necessary physiological activities. Though no specific frequency is deemed healthy and compulsory, defecating as frequently as possible is crucial. An individual must defecate frequently as it improves the gut, especially colon health.

Pooping regularly also reduces the risk of constipation and food retention in the gastrointestinal tract. Developing inflammation in the gut. Retention of food in the abdomen may predispose an individual to inflammation. It promotes the growth of harmful microorganisms that can destroy the body's beneficial organisms and inhibit communication through the brain-gut axis. If you find it challenging to defecate regularly, consider increasing the fibre content of your diet by eating foods like sweet potatoes, avocados, and whole grains such as barley, beans, broccoli, apples, bananas, etc.

Maintaining a Healthy Weight
Obesity is a steadily growing menace worldwide, and it has been implicated in the development of numerous life-threatening medical conditions such as diabetes, cardiovascular diseases, etc. Therefore, an individual must strive to maintain a healthy weight. Regarding the vagus nerve, research has shown that obesity and gut inflammation can impair vagus nerve function and adversely affect the brain-gut axis. Individuals struggling with obesity endeavour to lose weight by developing practical habits to help achieve long-term weight loss.

Endeavour to increase your daily activities, mainly if your line of work entails sitting at a place throughout the day. Aim to move around at least every hour for approximately 10 minutes to help improve circulation and alleviate the adverse effects caused by a sedentary lifestyle. Avoid eating late at night by aiming to have your dinner before 8 pm. Also, consider where you eat. Do not eat in front of the television because it can be distracting, causing you to overeat. Instead, find a place to sit, relax and eat while chewing slowly, as this would help you get filled more.

Rest and Sleep

The adequate amount of hours an individual should sleep ranges from 6-8 pm, according to medical experts; therefore, try to get proper rest and sleep daily. Also, strive to keep stress to a minimum. Engage in your hobbies and favourite activities that help you relax when stressed. If you still struggle to lose or maintain a healthy weight, please consult your medical doctor to understand the cause of weight gain and draft an appropriate program to help you achieve a healthy weight.

Fasting

One of the healthy habits medical experts advise individuals to develop is fasting. Not only does it help one lose and maintain an ideal weight, boosts cognitive function, protects one from developing obesity-associated chronic diseases, and reduces inflammation. Fasting is a physiological, natural stimulant of vagal-mediated pathways on the vagus nerve. It increases heart rate variability and breaks the digestive tract from digestion. This break causes the body's metabolism to reduce, stimulating the parasympathetic vagal response to this. The good thing about fasting is you do not have to fast for long periods to see results.

1 6

FOODS TO EAT TO HELP YOUR VAGUS NERVE

Activating the Vagus nerve through practices such as yoga, tai chi and singing can help to reduce inflammation and improve overall health.

ood is an essential component of human life, a necessity that can not be done without it. There is a famous saying that you are what you eat; hence, what you take in is what sustains your body. This shows that maintaining a healthy eating practice and lifestyle is paramount for an individual to live a healthy and prolonged life. You may be wondering how eating fit affects your vagus nerve; hence, we will discuss how eating healthy foods and maintaining healthy eating habits benefit the vagus nerve.

One of the significant causes of vagus nerve damage and decreased stimulation is chronic diseases and infections. Some conditions, like diabetes and hypothyroidism, have a dietary basis. For example, the increased consumption of high-calorie, sugary, or highly processed foods may predispose an individual to diabetes and obesity. Also, inadequate consumption of foods rich in iodine may predispose an individual to thyroid dysfunction, such as hypothyroidism. Some of these chronic disease conditions, such as obesity and cancer, may also become complicated and require surgery which increases the risk of vagus nerve damage during the surgery.

Hence, this emphasizes the need to eat healthy, nutrient-dense foods daily. Some of the foods that would benefit and improve vagal tone include

Foods Rich in Choline

Choline is an essential nutrient required in the human body. It is majorly obtained from dietary sources; hence, an individual's diet must include foods rich in choline to facilitate the synthesis of the neurotransmitter acetylcholine. Choline is a precursor to acetylcholine, the parasympathetic nervous system's primary neurotransmitter, enabling the vagus nerve to perform its functions. Hence, consuming more of these foods may help improve vagal tone.

Choline can be found in several food sources such as red beef, liver, turkey, kidney, pork, chicken breast, fish like salmon, caviar, cod, shrimp, tilapia, dairy products, and eggs. For individuals on vegetarian or plant-based diets, there are varieties of food sources, such as

- Fruits like apples, bananas, mangoes, avocados, berries e.t.c
- Cruciferous vegetables such as cauliflower, Brussels, broccoli, cabbage, kimchi,
- Whole grains and nuts such as almonds, lima beans, quinoa, peanuts
- Legumes such as kidney beans, peas like chickpeas, green peas e.t.c
- Potatoes, especially red potatoes
- Soy foods like tofu and edamame.

In addition to improving vagal tone, consuming foods rich in choline provides numerous benefits to the individual. Choline is needed to synthesize acetylcholine, essential in regulating memory, mood, and intelligence. Hence, scientists are inventing new methods of harnessing its potential to improve long-term cognitive health and reduce the risk of developing conditions like Alzheimer's disease.

Omega-3 Fatty Acids

Omega-3 fatty acids are essential to the vagus nerve as well as the overall health of an individual. The human body is unable to produce its omega-3 fatty acids. Therefore, these substances must be obtained from food consumed and supplements. Omega-3 acids are essential in cell functioning throughout the body, especially on receptors in cell membranes and nerve cells. Omega-3 fatty acids improve vagal tone and heart rate variability- a state of balance in the heart that is appropriately responsive to sympathetic and parasympathetic nervous stimulation. Omega-3 fatty acids also rapidly increase the repair rate in a damaged nerve.

In addition to improving vagal tone, omega-3 fatty acids stimulate the production of hormones that help regulate heart and blood function, which can help prevent heart disease and stroke. Some studies also show that omega-3 acids can help control chronic inflammatory diseases, like lupus erythematosus and rheumatoid arthritis, which could predispose an individual to vagus nerve damage.

Foods rich in omega-3 fatty acids include

- Fish like sardine, cod liver oil, caviar, mackerel, herrings, salmon e.t.c
- Seeds and nuts like chia seeds, walnuts, flax seeds
- Legumes like soybeans
- Eggs
- Meat such as beef, lamb, mutton e.t.c
- Dairy products like milk
- Fruits like blueberries and avocado
- Vegetables such as Brussels sprouts and spinach.

Other functions of omega-3 fatty acids include stimulation of proper brain development and health of the fetus during pregnancy and early life, improving eye health, prevention of cancer, helping to fight depression e.t.c

Foods Rich in Tryptophan

Tryptophan is an essential amino acid to build muscles and produce bodily enzymes and neurotransmitters. It is termed crucial because the body can not make it. Hence it must be obtained from the diet. Dietary tryptophan is obtained and metabolized in the gut, and research has shown that it may assist cells in the brain and spinal cord to control inflammation, which may impair the gut-brain axis via the vagal messenger pathway. Hence, tryptophan has anti-inflammatory effects that reduce the risk of vagus nerve damage due to chronic inflammatory diseases.

Foods rich in tryptophan include

- Dairy products such as milk (particularly whole milk), cheese, and yoghurt
- Vegetables like spinach, sunflower seeds, watercress, pumpkin seeds, mushrooms, broccoli, and peas
- Legumes like soybeans
- Eggs
- Seeds and nuts like peanuts, cashews, pistachios, and almonds
- Fruits such as bananas, plantains, pineapple, kiwi fruit, plums, and tomatoes
- Meat such as chicken, turkey, fish, pork, and salmon.

Foods Rich in Zinc

Research has shown that the trace mineral zinc is essential to numerous metabolic processes, including optimal vagus nerve. However, many individuals need this critical mineral in their diet. The body cannot store zinc for future use; hence, it should be consumed adequately in the diet. Studies have shown that zinc increases and maintains the optimal vagal tone. In addition, zinc also helps to support the immune system hence, reducing the risk of developing chronic diseases that could damage the vagus nerve deal with other mental disorders, such as depression and repair damaged body tissues.

Foods rich in zinc include:

- Seafood like oysters, lobsters, crabs, shrimps, mussels
- Meat such as chicken, beef, pork, lamb
- Eggs
- Dark Chocolate
- Whole Grains such as quinoa, wheat, rice
- Seeds and Nuts like almonds, cashew, pine nuts, peanuts, squash, pumpkin, and sesame seeds
- Dairy products like milk and cheese
- Legumes such as chickpeas and lentils.

Foods Rich in Magnesium

Magnesium is another vital mineral to optimize many physiological processes, including regulating muscular activities and blood sugar levels. It is also crucial in regulating the nervous system, especially the vagus nerve. Magnesium is essential for optimal vagus nerve stimulation and transmission of impulses to and fro the brain and organs.

Foods rich in magnesium include:

- Fruits like avocado, bananas, pineapples, figs, kiwis, guavas,
- Seeds and nuts like almonds, flax seeds, cashew, pumpkin seeds, chia seeds
- Soyfoods like tofu and edamame
- Whole grains like wheat, buckwheat, barley, and oats
- Eggs
- Leafy green vegetables like spinach, kale, swiss chard, collard greens, mustard greens
- Legumes like black beans, lentils, chickpeas, and kidney beans
- Fish such as salmon and mackerel
- Dark Chocolate
- Dairies like milk and yoghurt.

In addition, magnesium also improves bone health, improves bowel movements, helps fight depression, reduces the risk of developing chronic diseases like cardiovascular disease, reduces stress, and enables you to sleep better.

Foods Rich in Vitamin C

Vitamin C, ascorbic acid, can be considered an essential vitamin that the body can not do. It is required in almost everything that happens in the human body, from the growth and development of the body to the absorption of other nutrients and maintenance of the immune system. Vitamin C helps maintain the integrity and optimal functioning of the nervous system. It increases the stimulation and ability of the vagus nerve to respond to pressure variations. It stimulates the synthesis and release of acetylcholine which is the neurotransmitter that helps the vagus nerve perform its functions.

Foods rich in vitamin C include:

Fruits like oranges, Kakadu plums, strawberries, guavas, mangoes, grapefruits, lemons, blackcurrant, cantaloupe

Vegetables include kale, brussels sprouts, spinach, cauliflower, tomatoes, cabbage, broccoli, and bell peppers.

In addition, vitamin C also helps improve cognitive function as you age, reduces the risk of developing chronic diseases such as hypertension and cardio-vascular diseases, boosts immunity, and has anti-ageing properties due to its antioxidant function.

Foods to Avoid To Improve Vagal Tone

To improve and maintain a healthy vagal tone, avoiding unhealthy foods like highly processed foods, fatty foods, sugary foods and drinks, and high carbs and calories is essential. These foods are addictive and cause the brain to crave more by stimulating dopamine associated with pleasure and reward.

Sugar and highly processed foods have been linked to an improved risk of developing inflammatory diseases and cancer. Instead, eat whole, nutrient-dense foods, incorporating the abovementioned examples. If you are hungry between meals, instead of sugary or processed foods, have a healthy snack, like fruit, nuts, hard-boiled eggs, baked sweet potatoes or edamame.

This fact will give you more energy than packaged products. If you struggle with maintaining mindful and healthy eating habits, experts advise keeping a food journal to help you develop a healthy diet and eating pattern.

17

FREQUENTLY ASKED QUESTIONS ON
THE VAGUS NERVE

The Vagus nerve is the bridge between the brain and the gut, playing a crucial role in regulating digestion and gut health.

his section aims to provide quick and concise answers to many people's questions about the vagus nerve.

What is Vagus Nerve?

The vagus nerve also can be related to the wandering nerve, is a nerve comprising motor and sensory parts that provide most of the parasympathetic input to the gastrointestinal system, the motor fibres of the larynx and pharynx to the heart, and sensory fibres to the external acoustic meatus and meninges.

The 10th cranial nerve is a pair of Left and right Vagal nerves that perform unique involuntary functions like heart rate and digestion. This pair of nerves contain 75% of your parasympathetic nervous system's nerve fibres, which transport information between your digestive system, brain, and heart.

What are the sensory Ganglia of the Vagus Nerve?

The vagus nerve has two sensory ganglia: the superior and the inferior.

The superior ganglion is placed in the jugular foramen, where the vagus nerve exits the skull. It is smaller and proximal to the inferior ganglion of the vagus nerve.

The superior ganglion comprises neurons that innervate the poster-inferior surface of the external auditory canal, the concha of the auricle, and the postero-inferior surface of the tympanic membrane all through the auricular branch of the vagus nerve. It also contains neurons that can innervate part of the dura mater, where the posterior cranial is through the meningeal branch of the vagus nerve.

Conversely, the inferior ganglion is more significant and below the vagus nerve's superior ganglion. The superior ganglion is also placed in the jugular foramen in which the vagus nerve exits the skull, and a majority of neurons in the inferior ganglion provide sensory innervation to several body organs, including gastrointestinal tracts, the taste buds, the heart, respiratory and abdominal organs like the urinary bladder. The inferior ganglion has two branches: the pharyngeal nerve and the superior laryngeal nerve.

Where is the Vagus Nerve Located?

The vagus nerve is originated in the brain and exits via the medulla oblongata of the lower brainstem, from which it branches out in multiple directions. It extends from its origin in the brainstem and, from there, moves through the neck, the thorax, and down to the abdomen. It is a pair of nerves originating from the medulla oblongata's left and right sides. The left vagus nerve moves down the left side of the body, while the right vagus nerve moves down the right side.

What is Vasovagal Syncope?

The vagus nerve induces heart muscles that help slow heart rate. Vasovagal syncope happens when the sympathetic division dilates the blood vessels in the leg, and the vagal nerve overreacts, which can lead to a quick drop in blood pressure and heart rate. Ultimately, it results in dizziness or fainting.

Some factors which can trigger this include anxiety, pregnancy, extreme heat, emotional stress, and pain. However, these symptoms are only triggers and may be no exact cause of the problem. Apart from fainting, an individual may experience nausea, excessive sweating, tunnel vision, or ear ringing. Vasovagal syncope can be prevented by drinking lots of fluids and avoiding quick and sudden movements.

What is the Effect of Alcohol on the Vagus Nerve?

The vagus nerve is distributed throughout the body, which includes the heart, lungs, guts, and liver. It prevents inflammation in these organs by releasing acetylcholine (ACh) onto nicotinic receptors (nAChRs) of the alpha7- subtype. Apart from their presence in inflammatory cells, the alpha7-nAChRs are also present in cell bodies of the vagus in the CNS, which brings about neuroprotection and vagal activation. Alcohol intake inhibits alpha7-nAChRs, and brings about vagal neuropathy, thus jeopardizing the anti-inflammatory effects of the vagus nerve. It is essential to know that alcohol reduces cardiac vagal tone.

How are Vagus Nerve Disorders Diagnosed?

Any of these tests can be employed to help diagnose vagal nerves disorders:

- Endoscopy or X-rays - this test will tell if you have an intestinal or stomach blockage
- An echocardiogram will help take a closer look at your heart and surrounding blood vessels. It is an ultrasound of the heart to assess heart function.
- Computed Tomography (CT) scan or magnetic resonance imaging (MRI) can also be used.
- In chapter four of this book, you can find other methods to diagnose a vagus nerve disorder.

How can I Increase my Vagal Tone?

The vagus nerve is connected to the muscles located at the back of the throat and vocal cords, so engaging in activities triggers these muscles and stimulates your vagus nerve. These activities include gargling, chanting, singing, and humming and have been shown to increase vagal tone.

Getting regular massages or performing self-massage also does well to help vagal activity and improve vagal tone. Additionally, cold-water immersion may help relieve stress by directing blood flow to your brain and slowing your heart rate.

Probiotics like lactobacillus and Bifidobacterium have improved vagal tone and stimulation. Omega-3s are great foods that can help with improving vagal tone. Read chapters 5 to 15 of this book to learn more about these exercises listed.

Can a Weak Vagus Nerve Cause Digestive Issues?

Your gut is made up of the small and large intestines. The vagus nerve connects your core to the brain and plays a vital role in maintaining intestinal homeostasis, regulating food intake, satiety, and modulation of inflammation. During digestion, the vagus nerve recognizes changes in the microbiota in your intestines and transmits this information to your brain, and the brain immediately sends back the correct response. So if your vagus nerve is weak, the nerve can't effectively foster communication between the body and the brain, contributing to digestive disorders.

Does Vagus Neuropathy Cause Refractory Chronic Cough?

The hypersensitivity of the vagal afferent nerves causes refractory chronic cough. A vagus nerve disorder can change the afferent branches of the reflex laryngeal, and various stimuli, such as acid, can trigger cough symptoms.

Does Vagus Nerve Disorder Cause Low Stomach Acidity?

The vagus nerve is involved in regulating gastrin release and gastric acid secretion. Low stomach acidity is partially a result of vagus nerve disorder. Conditions that are related to low stomach acidity are inflammatory bowel diseases such as gastroparesis (stomach paralysis), Crohn's, ulcerative colitis (UC), gastroesophageal reflux disease (GERD), and heartburn.

Does Vagal Nerve Disorder Cause Gastroparesis?

Gastroparesis is when your stomach can't empty itself of food as usual. A healthy vagus nerve tightens or contracts the muscles of your abdomen to facilitate food movement through your digestive tract. Damage to the vagus nerve can prevent your stomach and intestine muscles from working as they should, thereby stopping food from moving into your intestine from your belly. Vagal nerve damage like this can result from abdominal surgery, scleroderma, diabetes, and viral infections.

Is the Vagus Nerve Responsible for Coughing?

The sensory nerves stimulate the afferents in the vagus nerve, which signals the medulla located in the brainstem to initiate the cough reflex. The medulla then sends signals back through the vagus nerve to the muscles between your ribs and diaphragm, instructing them to contract.

Can Vagus Nerve Stimulation Help in Spinal Cord Injury Recovery?

Vagus nerve stimulation (VNS) involves using a biomedical device that transmits moderate electrical currents to the brain through the vagus nerve. It helps control the autonomic nervous system, which is essential post spinal cord injury. VNS won't treat your spinal cord injury (SCI) but can boost your mental and physical health, putting your body in the best condition for recovery. Depression is a secondary complication experienced after SCI, and VNS is an FDA-approved treatment. VNS also boosts microglial M2 polarization by regulating α7nAChR to reduce neuroinflammation, thus improving motor function recovery after SCI.

Can Vagus Nerve Stimulation Help Patients with Epilepsy?

When Seizures persist after trying at least two prescribed anti-seizure medications, then it is considered drug-resistant epilepsy. Additional medications cannot control this epilepsy, but alternative non-drug therapy should be considered.

VNS Therapy can lead to fewer and shorter seizures and better recovery after seizures. It is an add-on neuromodulation treatment made specifically for people with drug-resistant epilepsy who are four years of age and older with partial-onset seizures.

VNS Therapy is a bioelectronic device surgically inserted under the skin in the chest and to the left vagus nerve located within the neck. It is programmed to administer mild electrical signals to the brain using the vagus nerve to prevent convulsions before they start and stop them.

Does Vagus nerve disorder cause GERD?

Gastroesophageal Reflux Disease (GERD) or chronic acid reflux is a disorder that arises partly due to Vagus nerve disorder. It is a condition whereby acid-containing content in your stomach leaks back up into your oesophagus because a valve at the end of your oesophagus (the lower oesophagal sphincter) doesn't close properly after the food arrives in your stomach, thus leading to the acid flowing back through your oesophagus into your throat and mouth.

Conclusion

In summary, the vagus nerve is an essential part of the human body that can be exercised to improve your overall health. The exercises outlined in this book have been shown to improve overall health and life quality for those who practice them regularly.

CONCLUSION

The candle is not destroyed when another candle lights it.

I am thankful you've taken some time and read through my book. I hope it has inspired and enlightened you to take control of your health.

Once you have a better understanding of the structure of the parasympathetic nervous system as well as the degree to that it VN communicates, it is yours to boost its performance and improve your well-being. For some, these methods and strategies can have profound effects which will significantly enhance your digestion, energy, and inflammation. It could be the beginning of your journey to better health for others.

Tell people around you - family, friends, and loved ones who may want to know that there is a solution to the reasons that may be making them sick.

If you have significant improvements after implementing sure of the easy changes by this publication, continue to keep going strong and develop better habits. If you require someone to help you throughout the process, it's a good thing and not something to be shameful. Find forward-thinking health providers who don't follow the conventional approach to medical practices. Find someone who can help you in a way that genuinely cares about you as a person and guide you in determining the root of your problems.

I am genuinely thankful for each one of you. I wish you the very best in your journey.

In summary, the vagus nerve is an important part of the human body that can be exercised to improve your overall health. The exercises outlined in this book have been proven to improve overall health and quality of life for those who practice them regularly.

THANK YOU

Thank you for taking the time to read this book. We hope that it has been informative and helpful to you. We understand that some of the material may have been challenging to understand, but we believe that by reading this book again and again, you will be able to fully grasp the concepts and gain the most benefit from it. We recommend reading it at least once a month to keep the information fresh in your mind. As a token of our appreciation for your dedication, we have included a special surprise for you at the end of the book.

A guide to "Discover How To Become Whole Mentally, Physically, and Spiritually". Thank you for your support and we hope that you continue to find value in our work.

THE POLYVAGAL THEORY

The Polyvagal Theory

INTRODUCTION

INTRODUCTION

Welcome to the polyvagal theory! Here, you will learn just how your vagus nerve affects your emotions and how much control you can have over it.

If you are reading this, it is most likely because you are interested in learning how our brains work in conjunction with our bodies or maybe just curious about the world around you. No matter your reason for reading this book, we want to ensure that you're getting a solid introduction to the polyvagal theory.

The world that we live in is increasingly defined by the things we do. We are urged to be more productive, active, and engaged with our environment. But what does this mean for us? It means that we don't have time to sit still and relax. It means that we're constantly on the go, always doing something -whether it be work or play- instead of just being. It means that we spend so much of our lives afraid of being judged, failing, hurt, or disappointed by others that we become tense and anxious in response to those fears.

This is why so many people suffer from anxiety disorders: because they can't stop the stress response from happening when they feel anxious. They need their brains to tell them over and over again that everything is OK -even though it isn't- so they can continue with their busy lives without having to deal with the full implications of their actions. This constant stress can lead to health problems like heart disease and hypertension, as well as mental health issues like depression and PTSD (post-traumatic stress disorder).

The good news is that there is an alternative way of thinking about how our brains work: the polyvagal theory!

So what is it? The polyvagal theory was developed by Stephen W. Porges and first stated at his address to the Society of Psychophysiological Research at a meeting that was held in Atlanta, Georgia, in 1994. It explains how our nervous system evolved over time, specifically how our ancestors' nervous systems worked, and why they might have been so successful at staying alive.

The polyvagal theory is a scientific approach to understanding how people work together. It's based on the idea that our nervous system has two separate but equally important parts -the first is the sympathetic nervous system, which triggers flight or fight when we're in danger. The second part of our nervous system is called the parasympathetic nervous system, which keeps us calm and focused when there's no danger.

Simply put, sympathetic impulses are associated with arousal or intense feelings like anger and fear; parasympathetic impulses, on the other hand, are associated with rest, relaxation, and sleepiness. The theory also suggests that these two types of impulses work together to keep us safe from danger -if we experience an emotion that triggers both our sympathetic and parasympathetic systems.

According to the polyvagal theory, humans are naturally wired to be able to switch between these two systems, depending on what they need at that moment. For example, if you're walking down a busy street and someone bumps into you, your sympathetic nervous system will kick in and make you feel startled, angry, or afraid. But if you think about it for a second and realize that the person probably didn't mean any harm by bumping into you, your parasympathetic system will kick in and calm you down. This is especially helpful when managing stress -you can use your parasympathetic system to help you relax or even fall asleep whenever needed!

The polyvagal theory is a new way of thinking about the brain and human behavior. It says that we are not just hard-wired for fight or flight but also for play, relaxation, and connection. The theory tries to explain how these functions work together in our bodies and how they can be used to improve our health and wellness.

The vagal nerves are important because they regulate how much oxygen reaches your brain and how much sugar (glucose) gets there. This is because when you're stressed out or anxious, your heart rate increases, and your blood pressure increases. And this can affect how well those two things are regulated: if your blood vessels aren't getting enough oxygen, your brain won't get enough sugar, making it harder for your body to function normally.

So what does that mean? Basically, if you want to feel more calm and relaxed, you have to make sure that you keep those two things going well: you have to be sure that your heart is regulating itself well so that it's delivering enough blood with enough oxygen, and you have to be sure that your brain has enough sugar so that it can function normally.

In essence, the polyvagal theory is a way to understand how these two systems work together, to understand better how they can function independently from one another, and how they can be used in healthy ways. So what does that all mean?

Well, for starters, it means that you don't have to rely on your sympathetic nervous system alone when you need to calm down -you can also use other methods! And it also means that instead of having one group of nerves controlling all aspects of your body's response, you have two groups of nerves working together. So not only can you relax when needed without relying solely on your sympathetic nervous system, but this relaxed state can help keep your sympathetic nervous system functioning properly. Without further ado, let's dig in.

1

─────────────

WHAT IS THE POLYVAGAL THEORY

$\mathcal{T}$he polyvagal theory is a model of emotional regulation that explains how the nervous system contributes to the experience of emotion. It was developed by Dr. Stephen Porges in 1979 and has since been used to understand a wide range of disorders, including post-traumatic stress disorder (PTSD), depression, anxiety, and eating disorders.

The theory posits that our nervous system is made up of three different parts: an autonomic nervous system (ANS), a somatic nervous system (SNS), and an enteric nervous system (ENS). The ANS regulates our body's basic functions like breathing, digestion, heart rate, etc., the SNS regulates our muscles, and the ENS regulates our internal organs.

The first two systems are responsible for our automatic behaviors - the way we move when we're not thinking about them or trying to control them - and they're largely unconscious. The ENS, on the other hand, is conscious and voluntary; it can be activated by thoughts like "I feel anxious" or "I want to eat badly."

The theory suggests that this third system plays a role in regulating emotions because it is capable of influencing both autonomic and somatic processes that occur unconsciously throughout the body. It also states that our brains have two separate but complementary systems for processing emotions: one system is associated with the primitive, fast-acting fight-or-flight response, whereas the other is associated with more complex processes such as social bonding and emotional responsiveness.

Since its establishment, the polyvagal theory has been applied to many different areas of psychology and neuroscience research, including how people experience their own emotions, how they communicate with others, how they experience the emotions of other people, how they respond to stress; and even how they respond to trauma or physical injury.

This theory also recognizes that there are three different parts of the nervous system that are responsible for controlling bodily functions, including breathing and heart rate. These three parts are called the sympathetic nervous system, enteric nervous system, and vagal nerve.

Your sympathetic nervous system (SNS) is responsible for keeping you alive by increasing your heart rate and breathing rate to keep you from freezing in cold weather. If it does not work properly or if there is any sort of damage to this part of your body, then you may die from hypothermia. The enteric nervous system does not receive as much attention from researchers but is still very important in many ways. This part of your body controls motor movement and digestion, which can be very important when you are trying to survive on your own without anyone else who can help you with food or water supplies.

Finally, there is the vagal nerve which controls most other bodily functions, including heart rate and breathing which allows you to survive in almost any environment even if there isn't enough oxygen available around you due to environmental factors like weather conditions or altitude changes.

Moving further, let us establish that the nervous system comprises many parts, including the brain, spinal cord, and peripheral nerves. The central nervous system (CNS) controls voluntary motor activity, while the peripheral nervous system (PNS) controls involuntary motor activity such as breathing.

The PNS includes both sympathetic and parasympathetic divisions; these two systems are responsible for controlling our fight-or-flight response. The sympathetic nervous system ensures the body is prepared for fight or flight; it makes us more alert and responsive to danger. This part of the nervous system is what we're used to seeing in people who are anxious or afraid. It is activated by stressors like fear or pain and can cause us to freeze or flee from the source of danger in order to protect ourselves from harm. It also causes us to experience a surge in blood pressure and heart rate in order to prepare us for action.

The parasympathetic nervous system is designed to help us return to a calm state after an emergency response. It slows down our heart rate, dilates our pupils, lowers blood pressure, increases relaxation hormones like oxytocin, and increases digestive functions like salivation. This part of the nervous system is what we're used to seeing in people who are calm or relaxed after an emergency has passed, and it is activated by non-stressors like rest and relaxation.

Both of these systems work closely together as a team throughout our lives, but some people have more difficulty regulating them than others due to genetics or other factors such as childhood trauma or abuse.

The polyvagal theory is a way to understand how the nervous system works and how it can affect our emotional health. It suggests that there's more going on than just these two systems working together -the two systems can actually influence each other! It is possible that if one part of the nervous system were activated while another was inhibited, this would negatively affect emotional health because it would increase the activation of one set of nerves while inhibiting another.

BACKGROUND TO THE POLYVAGAL THEORY

The polyvagal theory has been around for almost 30 years and was first described by neuroscientist Stephen Porges in 1994. It is a theory that explains how our brains are able to regulate our emotions and behaviors.

His work was inspired by several other theories, including Harry Harlow's "abandoned baby" experiments and John Bowlby's attachment theory -which suggested that early childhood experiences are critical to later adult behavior. Porges' paper "The Polyvagal Theory: Neurophysiological Foundations of Emotions Relevant to Social Interactions" provided an overview of his ideas on how a person's physiological state can influence their emotional state.

This theory is based on research done in the 1990s, which explored how the brain's nervous system can be divided into two parts: the sympathetic nervous system, which controls our body's fight-or-flight response, and the parasympathetic nervous system, which assists us relax and calm down.

The sympathetic nervous system is controlled by the amygdala -a small area of the brain in the middle of your forebrain that is responsible for emotional responses, behavior, and motivation- while the parasympathetic system is controlled by a different part of your brain called the vagus nerve.

Porges divided human emotions into four categories: social engagement, such as smiling or laughter; protective pursuit, such as fleeing from danger; aggressive response, such as anger; and affiliative behaviors, such as touching or hugging others. He believed these categories were linked to specific physiological responses such as increased heart rate.

In his research, Porges found that both sympathetic and parasympathetic nervous systems are involved in emotional regulation. The sympathetic nervous system comes alive when we become aroused or excited, and it increases our heart rate, blood pressure, and respiration. The parasympathetic nervous system then takes over and helps us return to baseline by slowing down our heart rate, blood pressure, and breathing.

Porges also found that the primary function of the vagus nerve is to connect the brain to the immune system. This means that when someone has a strong connection between their emotional state and their immune system functioning well, they can better regulate their emotional responses in stressful situations. For example, if someone is angry or scared, but their vagus nerve is working properly, they will be able to vent those feelings without triggering an increase in inflammatory responses like cortisol release or an attack on the tissue around their heart, known as myocardial infarction.

Over time, this theory has evolved to accommodate research, and even more facts have been established about the vagus nerve than there were 30 years ago. Going forward, let us take a look at some of the basic principles the polyvagal theory stands for.

CONTROVERSIES SURROUNDING THE POLYVAGAL THEORY

The Polyvagal Theory is over two decades old, and it suggests that the vagus nerve is the key to social communication. This theory was developed and promulgated by Dr. Stephen Porges, and it is currently one of the most widely-used concepts in neuroscience.

However, there are some controversies surrounding this theory. One controversy is that there's no evidence to support it. The second controversy is that it's not widely accepted by other scientists because it's not well-documented or peer-reviewed.

The first controversy is whether or not the polyvagal theory is accurate. The theory suggests that humans have three separate branches of the vagus nerve, and each branch has a different function. One branch is responsible for mobilizing our bodies to fight or flee from danger; another controls blood pressure and heart rate during periods of stress, and the third helps us regulate our digestion and other internal mechanisms.

It is believed that if you can train yourself to activate these different branches of your vagus nerve, you will be able to manage stress and anxiety in your life better, as well as improve your overall health. However, some researchers are of the strong opinion that this is not a complete picture of human behavior and physiology. They argue that there are other factors involved in stress management and anxiety reduction than just activating the vagus nerve. Some researchers also argue that the polyvagal theory does not account for differences between men and women when it comes to managing stress or anxiety.

Also, some researchers think that it's too simplistic to say that the nervous system is divided into two parts: sympathetic and parasympathetic. They believe that it's more accurate to say that there are three parts: sympathetic, parasympathetic, and the enteric nervous system (ENS). The ENS has its own independent nervous system, which can be considered a third branch of the autonomic nervous system.

According to this theory, the parasympathetic branch controls digestion and other internal functions like breathing and heart rate, while the sympathetic branch helps you respond quickly to danger by speeding up your heart rate and increasing blood flow through your muscles. However, some scientists believe that both branches of the autonomic nervous system work together in response to stressors—for example, when someone experiences intense pain due to an injury or burns from fire (which would cause a surge in adrenaline), both branches would activate at once.

Another controversy is whether or not we should use terms like "**fight-or-flight**" when describing how our bodies react during stressful situations like emergencies or emergencies and whether those terms are even accurate descriptions of what happens when we feel.

2

PRIMARY PRINCIPLES OF POLYVAGAL
THEORY

*T*he Polyvagal Theory emphasizes two important functions: vagal tone and heart rate variability (HRV). Vagal tone is the degree of activation of your vagus nerve, which runs from your brain stem down through your chest and abdomen. When you're in a state of high vagal tone -when your nerve is firing off signals at a strong rate- you'll feel more relaxed and calm than when you're in a state of low vagal tone, in which case you're likely to feel tense or stressed out. Also, since your vagus nerve will be less active, you'll be more likely to experience feelings of anxiety.

HRV refers to how fast your heart rate varies from beat to beat; low HRV means the heart rate goes up and down quickly with each beat, while high HRV means that the beats are spread out over longer periods of time.

Here are some of the most basic principles of the polyvagal theory:

THE FUNCTION OF THE AUTONOMIC STATE AS AN 'INTERVENING VARIABLE

According to the Polyvagal Theory, the physiological state is a fundamental component of emotion or mood rather than merely a correlate. The theory states that our perception and assessment of environmental cues are influenced by the autonomic state, which acts as an intervening variable.

The same cues will be reflexively interpreted as neutral, favorable, or threatening, depending on the physiological state. Functionally, a change in state will modify access to various brain regions and facilitate either social interaction or defensive behaviors like fight-or-flight or shutdown.

The theory emphasizes that the physiological state greatly influences a person's behavior and mental state, including their ability to learn and remember, as well as their ability to feel, control emotions and socialize. It also emphasizes that a person's physiological state can also play a role in the outcome of any medical treatment they are given and their general state of health.

According to the Polyvagal Theory, stress is simply a persistent disturbance of homeostatic regulation. Temporary difficulties that the autonomic nervous system can quickly recover from are not stress, nor are they always the results of sympathetic-adrenal activation, which is necessary for increased metabolic activity linked to movement. As long as they are temporary, the autonomic nervous system can naturally adapt to support metabolic demands and, in no time, return to a state that sustains homeostatic processes. A defensive autonomic nervous system that is tuned in this way is capable of supporting hypervigilance and hypersensitivities while also jeopardizing the neural control of visceral organs.

FUNCTION OF THE VENTRAL VAGAL PATHWAYS AS A TRANSITORY VAGAL BRAKE

For many decades, sustained attention and mental effort were always measured by changes in heart rate variability (HRV). Besides, tons of research carried out across many laboratories have shown that certain HRV indicators, such as respiratory sinus arrhythmia, were suppressed during forms of awareness, expectation, and exercise.

The ventral vagal pathway, according to the polyvagal theory, is identified as the structure underlying the vagal brake. Some recent research has shown the role of the recuperation of respiratory sinus arrhythmia as a vital indicator of social behavior and state control, thus leading to a hypothesis that the ventral vagal cardioinhibitory pathway is involved in both coregulation and self-regulation.

With the concept of the vagal brake, the measurement of the changes in heart rate variability during mental and physical challenges could be comprehended from a neurobiological perspective.

AUTONOMIC REACTIVITY AS AN EVOLUTIONARY RESPONSE

The polyvagal theory states that when challenges are encountered, the autonomic state moves through an evolutionary sequence. A hierarchy develops whereby newer responses inhibit older responses; this concept is known as dissolution, which was introduced by John Hughlings Jackson. Like that of many mammals, the human nervous system developed over time to ensure stability in safe environments, as well as survival in dangerous environments.

According to John Hughlings Jackson's construct of dissolution, "the higher nervous arrangements inhibit (or control), the lower, and thus when the higher are suddenly rendered functionless, the lower rise in activity." This means that the most recent responses are used first, and if they fail to provide safety for the body, then older responses are adapted.

Three stages of response have been developed gradually during human evolution and are largely involved in the functioning of our autonomic nervous system. These three responses form a hierarchy. When dealing with stress, the body typically uses the most advanced -the most recent- response, and if it does not work, the body immediately switches to an older response.

IMMOBILIZATION/FREEZE/SHUTDOWN

The polyvagal theory holds that parasympathetic immobilization is the most ancient and unevolved response to danger. Have you ever been in a situation -or seen it happen around you- where you are faced with a dangerous, possibly life-threatening situation and suddenly become frozen, numb, and unable to move? That was simply your body shutting down. Now, how does it work?

When the sympathetic system finds itself overwhelmed by a situation and unable to handle it, the autonomic nervous system automatically shuts down the body in a bid to self-preserve by conserving energy. While in a state of mobilization, the nervous system kicks into a heightened state which requires a lot of energy; immobilization seeks to reduce metabolism and save energy. This state can be likened to the state of "playing dead" that some animals exhibit.

When this happens, it is almost as though the parasympathetic system, instead of helping you slow down, kicks into overdrive, thus leading to a frozen state. This state is characterized by a ceasure of movement, reduced metabolism, reduced need to feed, and pain numbing. However, despite being immobilized, the sympathetic system is still sufficiently active enough to allow blood flow, maintain muscle tone, and, most importantly, maintain consciousness. This state is most common among people that have survived a highly traumatic event.

In extreme cases, the nervous system may totally collapse, leading to an over-activation of the dorsal (back) part of the vagus nerve, which subsequently leads to fainting. This explains why sometimes, a person immediately loses consciousness whenever they receive shocking news or find themselves in an unexpected situation. However, this state of a complete shutdown could prove very fatal because the brain does not receive enough oxygenated blood. So, instead of a total shutdown, the nervous system evolved and instead put us in a state of freeze.

MOBILIZATION/ FIGHT OR FLIGHT

Mobilization, which is also known as the fight or flight response, is a sympathetic reaction to certain circumstances, such as danger or shock. This response is mainly characterized by an increase in heart rate, perspiration, and a heightened state of stress and tension. In some cases, panic, anger, or anxiety may be experienced.

This simply signals that the body is activating the sympathetic nervous system to put up a fight against danger or to run from it. The fight-or-flight response prepares your body for immediate action by releasing hormones such as adrenaline and cortisol into your bloodstream. These hormones activate all major organs in your body, including your heart rate and respiration rate, sweating, muscle tension, and blood flow through your body.

In preparation, certain internal resources in the body, such as blood, are redirected from the digestive system to the extremities, which are the limbs and muscles, leading to the suspension of certain bodily functions. Additionally, the adrenal gland produces high levels of cortisol, which is known as the stress hormone. This explains why you may notice that when you are experiencing a lot of stress or anxiety, you might find yourself having digestive issues or having regular bouts of colds, as cortisol reduces the strength of the immune system.

Because the body is consuming a whole lot of resources and energy in this state, fatigue is undoubtedly going to set in after a while. According to the polyvagal theory, this response was the next to develop after the immobilization response, and it cannot be used simultaneously with other responses.

SOCIAL ENGAGEMENT / REST AND DIGEST

Social engagement is the most recent and evolved addition to the human hierarchy of responses to danger. This response is active via the ventral -front- part of the vagus nerve, unlike immobilization, which is activated through the dorsal part. Humans thrive best in a state of safety and rest; as a result, we naturally always want to be in this state unless faced with a threat.

The autonomic nervous system identifies a safe environment and responds to feelings of trust, safety, connection, calmness, and engagement, thus helping us build positive attachments. Unlike in the fight or flight state, normal bodily functions, such as digestion, are well regulated in the rest and digest state. Blood is present in the digestive system to support metabolism, and the immune system is optimized.

When faced with danger, this response attempts to negotiate and interact until a compromise that benefits both parties can be brokered. However, if this response fails, the nervous system automatically reverts to the fight or flight response, and if that one also fails, the immobilization is activated.

Traumatic experiences can disturb this system's reactions to danger and cooperative behaviors. A prolonged absence from this state of rest and social engagement can lead to a higher risk of death due to a weakened immune system and lack of interaction.

NEUROCONCEPTION AND THE AUTONOMIC STATE

Neuroconception is a system that is capable of instantly changing from one physiological state to another based on reflex. In humans, neuroconception is proposed to be launched by top-down pathways involving the parts of the brain that translate cues of danger and security. These cortical regions are perceptive to the deliberateness of body movements, such as voices, facial expressions, and gestures, and they can interpret these movements to either mean safety or danger. Following this interpretation, the nervous system will be signaled to produce the appropriate response to these movements.

Simply put, neuroconception deciphers and translates the supposed goal of movements and sounds from all living and non-living objects. This implies that with individuals who are familiar, neuro conception translated their voices and facial expressions into a positive interaction synonymous with a state of safety, while with individuals that are not familiar, neuro conception translates their voices and facial expressions, deducing whether they are friendly or hostile, and alerting the autonomic nervous system to act accordingly.

All living organisms have a type of neuro conception, regardless of how highly or lowly developed their nervous system is. However, among mammals, the capacity for neuroconception is highly developed, enabling them to reflexively respond to both threat and safety. You should know that neuroconception is more of a gut feeling than anything concrete.

COREGULATION AND NEUROCONCEPTION

The connection between coregulation and neuro conception is as follows: coregulation occurs when two individuals move together in a coordinated manner, such as when two people dance together or when they take turns playing musical instruments. Coregulation helps us understand what another person is feeling because it involves both mirroring their behavior and engaging in reciprocal interactions with them.

Coregulation is a process by which the nervous system communicates with other systems in the body to coordinate behavior. This is especially important for social interactions because, according to the polyvagal theory, we have different ways of responding to stress depending on whether we are interacting with someone we know or don't know.

Coregulation and neuroconception are two important concepts in polyvagal theory. Coregulation refers to the process of adapting one's behavior based on another person's actions. Neuroconception is the process by which a person's nervous system detects threats that can affect their behavior.

Coregulation is a key component of neuroconception, but it can also occur without being prompted by fear. For example, if you're having a conversation with someone and they suddenly start leaning forward or sitting back, you might automatically respond with a similar movement of your own body. This is coregulation because you are adapting your behavior based on theirs.

It's important to note that coregulation does not necessarily mean that one person is controlling another person's behavior; rather, it means that two people are working together to influence each other's actions.

3

TRAUMA ON THE NERVOUS SYSTEM

*T*he nervous system is a complex, delicate system that controls all of our body's functions, including breathing, muscle movement, heart rate, and blood pressure. This system is made up of the brain, spinal cord, and nerves and helps you sense things like touch, heat, and pain.

When the nervous system is traumatized, it can change in ways that make it more difficult to do routine tasks or live normally. This can happen when you have an injury or illness that affects your brain and spine or if you experience something that leaves you feeling frightened or overwhelmed.

When something traumatic happens to you -like an accident or injury- your brain goes through a series of steps to help you cope with it. This process is called trauma response, and it happens automatically in your body when you experience something stressful or frightening. But sometimes, trauma response can lead to problems with your nervous system if it continues for longer than expected or if you don't get proper treatment for whatever caused it in the first place.

Trauma can also affect other parts of your body, such as your muscles, bones, skin, and eyes. Trauma may also cause changes in your behavior and how you think about things; it is called post-traumatic stress disorder (PTSD).

Trauma isn't always caused by one incident: sometimes, it can be caused by many different events happening over time -like being bullied at school or your place of work- or by one event that happens over and over again -like experiencing abuse from one particular person.

The effects of trauma on the nervous system depend on various factors, such as:

1. The severity of the injury
2. The duration of injury
3. The type of injury sustained.

WHAT ARE THE EFFECTS OF TRAUMA ON THE NERVOUS SYSTEM?

Trauma can be physical or psychological, and it can be caused by a wide variety of factors. These factors may be physical, such as a blow to the head from a fall down a staircase or car accident, or they may be emotional, such as a divorce, sexual assault, or the loss of a loved one. In both cases, the trauma affects the brain and sends messages to the body, telling it that something is wrong. The body responds by producing chemicals called hormones that cause different reactions in various parts of the body.

Trauma can lead to problems with your nervous system if your nervous system is damaged by it. These problems include, but are not limited to:

HEADACHES (TENSION-TYPE HEADACHES)

Trauma is a common cause of headaches in adults, which are one of the most commonly reported problems after a traumatic event, such as car crashes or domestic violence. This ache is mostly characterized by pain in the head or face.

Headaches come in different kinds; they can be mild and short-lived or severe and long-lasting, depending on the type of injury sustained and its severity. They may also be accompanied by sensitivity to light or noise and sensitivity to smells, tastes, or touch.

In certain cases, headaches could be the result of injuries to the head or neck. In other cases, they may be related to anxiety and stress. Sometimes they are caused by an underlying medical condition that needs treatment, such as sinusitis, tension headaches, and migraines. But other than those, several other types of headaches can be caused by trauma.

The most common type of headache that results from trauma is a tension-type headache. This type of headache occurs when there is a muscle spasm in one or more areas of the neck. The muscles are tight and painful, causing pressure on the nerves in the neck which then leads to pain in other parts of the body.

Other examples of trauma-related headaches include:

Sinus headaches occur when pressure on the middle ear becomes painful due to fluid build-up or infection.

Migraine headaches: These are defined as severe headaches with no definite cause that last for more than four days and have been present for at least three months before treatment.

Aneurysm syndrome: This condition is characterized by an abnormal widening or bulging of arterial walls that may lead to rupture.

DIZZINESS/VERTIGO

This is usually very common amongst people who have just experienced trauma of any sort. It can be accompanied by a loss of balance, a false sense of spinning, light-headedness, unsteadiness, and a feeling of floating.

Dizziness has been reported as one of the most common neurological symptoms that occur after trauma. The dizziness may be caused by a disturbance in the balance system, which is located in the inner ear and brain. This can result from a hit to the head, whiplash, or even a low-speed car accident. Dizziness caused by trauma may be temporary or permanent. Temporary dizziness may occur within minutes of the event that caused it, while permanent dizziness may take months or years to develop.

Dizziness usually resolves within 24 to 48 hours of treatment. If it persists beyond this time, see your doctor for further evaluation.

SLEEP ISSUES (INSOMNIA)

It is a well established fact that sleep problems are common following trauma. In a study of post-traumatic stress disorder (PTSD) patients, insomnia was present in 86% of cases, and nightmares were present in 70% of cases. The most common complaint was difficulty falling asleep or staying asleep.

Insomnia may be brought on by traumatic memories of being attacked during the event or reliving the trauma, or it may be related to depression. Although insomnia can be caused by physical issues such as pain or excessive dreaming, mental health disorders such as depression, anxiety, and substance abuse disorders are among the most common causes of insomnia in people with PTSD.

For example, people suffering from PTSD, fully known as a post-traumatic stress disorder, often have trouble falling asleep and staying asleep. They may find themselves waking up earlier than usual in the morning because they are afraid that they will go back to their traumatic experiences -although they may not complain about it. As a result, they barely get enough sleep, which makes them feel tired during the day. All of these can ultimately lead to problems at work or school, such as trouble concentrating or irritability, and other health problems, such as headaches and stomach pain.

ANXIETY/DEPRESSION

Anxiety and depression are the most common mental health problems that people experience in response to trauma. Trauma can cause both anxiety and depression at the same time, or it may trigger just one of these conditions.

Depression and anxiety are both highly likely to be caused by trauma, but they're not the same thing. Let's take a quick look:

Anxiety

Anxiety is an incessant feeling of unease, worry, or nervousness, that can be mild or severe and varies from person to person. Anxiety is generally characterized by feelings of fear, apprehension, and worry to an excessive degree. They include generalized anxiety disorder (GAD), which involves persistent and excessive worry about many events in life. Worries may be based on fear of harm occurring to oneself or others and phobias, which involve extreme fear of specific objects, places, or situations such as heights, enclosed spaces, or flying on airplanes.

Panic disorder is majorly characterized by sudden episodes of intense fear, usually accompanied by physical symptoms, including shortness of breath, chest ache, and heart palpitations. People with panic disorder often have agoraphobia - the fear of being outside your home- which may involve avoiding situations where help isn't readily available if needed.

Anxiety may be triggered by a traumatic event or anticipation of a future traumatic experience. Anxiety is often characterized by physical symptoms such as increased heart rate and sweating, shaking, and shortness of breath. People who have so many anxiety disorders tend to worry excessively about possible threats and often have trouble controlling their fears. They may avoid situations that trigger fear or feel anxious even when they are not in danger.

Depression

Depression is another emotional disorder that involves feelings of sadness, worthlessness, and hopelessness for weeks or months at a time. The cause of depression can be caused by a wide range of things, including traumatic events, brain injury, genetic factors, drug use, and stress from other life events such as divorce or the death of a loved one.

Hyperarousal

Hyperarousal is a state in which a person's nervous system is in overdrive. This means that you are easily startled and may be jumpy or easily startled by loud noises and unexpected movements. This can happen after traumatic experiences, but it can also be a result of other types of stress. Hyperarousal can be a symptom of PTSD or other disorders such as depression and anxiety. Hyperarousal can also be an effect of trauma that occurs independently of PTSD or other disorders.

Hyperarousal is often described as feeling "on edge," "anxious," "fidgety," or "stressed." Hyperarousal may cause you to be easily startled, feel irritable and overwhelmed, have difficulty concentrating, and have trouble sleeping. You might also experience increased irritability and anger.

HYPERVIGILANCE AND PARANOIA

This is an extreme state of alertness that can cause you to feel like everything around you is dangerous, even when it's not. Hypervigilance and paranoia are mostly a result of trauma.

Hypervigilance is a condition in which the person experiences intense fear and anxiety. Hypervigilance is often associated with panic disorder. The hypervigilance can be triggered by a loud noise, an unexpected encounter with someone they don't know, or simply being in an unfamiliar environment.

Paranoia is the extreme distrust of others that leads to suspiciousness, distrustfulness, and suspiciousness. It may also include persecutory delusions. Paranoia can be triggered by an unexpected sound or event in the environment that takes away your control over your surroundings, for example, someone walking towards you on a busy street.

Hypervigilance and paranoia can be triggered by traumatic events that occur during or after the trauma. Hypervigilance is characterized by a heightened awareness of internal or external threats. Paranoia is characterized by an unreasonable belief that others are trying to hurt you or that they are harming you. The problem with hypervigilance is that it can become over-reliant on fear, causing problems for the individual who is constantly on alert for threats.

Dissociation

Dissociation is a psychological process by which the mind and body are separated, resulting in a loss of connection between them. It is a defense mechanism that allows the person to detach themselves from the pain of their trauma and emotions. It is often described as a "mental wall" that protects them from overwhelming feelings.

Dissociation is a normal response to trauma. In people who have experienced trauma, dissociation can be an adaptive response that helps them cope with the stress of the situation they find themselves in.

This happens when you disconnect from what's happening in the present moment, causing you to feel detached from reality or unable to remember what happened during the traumatic event. While this may be caused by external events, note that it is also a normal response to extreme stress. However, it can cause significant problems for the individual when it becomes chronic and habitual.

Dissociation can include:

- Flashbacks, where the memory of an event or experience is replayed in the present moment;
- Vivid and detailed imagery, such as visual images or sounds;
- Intrusive thoughts or intrusive memories that do not belong to you;
- Nightmares or bad dreams; and
- Difficulty staying focused on one task or thought.

HOW TO HEAL TRAUMA AND IMPROVE THE NERVOUS SYSTEM

Trauma has a deep effect on the nervous system, which can lead to lifelong symptoms and disorders. The nervous system is made up of nerves and brain cells, and when trauma occurs, it can affect the function of these tissues. In severe cases, the trauma can even cause damage to neurons in the brain or spinal cord, which can lead to long-term problems with memory, concentration, or motor skills.

Healing trauma is a complex process involving the nervous system, and this includes physical, emotional, and in some cases, spiritual methods. For example, you can use spiritual practices such as prayer and meditation to help you heal your emotional trauma. If you have a physical injury affecting your nervous system, you may also need to see a doctor for treatment.

When it comes to healing trauma, there are two main methods. The first and most common method is to talk about the trauma. This can be done through professional therapy, journaling, or just talking about the experience. The second method is to work on the physical symptoms of the trauma. Some people find that working on physical symptoms improves their mood and helps them feel more in control of their lives.

There are many different physical methods that can be used to heal trauma. Here are some of them:

Practice relaxation techniques: Relaxation techniques include breathing exercises, meditation, and massage therapy. They help reduce stress levels and increase blood flow to your brain and body, making you feel more relaxed and alert.

Exercise: Everyone, at one point in their lives, has carried out one form of exercise or the other. Even the simplest exercises, such as walking, can help improve circulation and reduces inflammation in your body. It also improves your mood by increasing endorphins (painkillers produced naturally).

Eat healthy foods: Eating nutritious foods helps prevent chronic conditions such as obesity, diabetes, and heart disease by improving digestion and metabolism. Healthy eating also reduces inflammation in your brain, which may help repair injuries from trauma.

Meditation: This is a powerful tool for healing both emotional and physical wounds. It helps you release any negative energy stored in your body and mind by using your imagination to focus on positive emotions such as peace or love. You may even want to try guided meditations if you want more direction or motivation during your sessions.

Massage therapy: This procedure uses pressure points on specific parts of the body to stimulate blood flow and lymphatic drainage (the natural process of removing toxins from your body). Massage therapists often combine this with various forms of stretching exercises to help increase flexibility and reduce stress levels in specific areas of the body.

4

THE VAGUS NERVE

*I*n the first book of this bundle, the vagus nerve was discussed in detail. However, seeing that the polyvagal theory gets its name from the vagus nerve, more light still needs to be shed on this vital part of the nervous system in this book. So, let's begin with the question - **what is the vagus nerve?**

The vagus nerve is a **group of nerves** that stem from the brain and descends through the neck. It is the longest nerve in the whole human body, with a total length of about 15 feet. It runs along the floor of the chest and abdomen, connecting to many different organs, including the head, neck, heart, lungs, and abdomen. It passes through the dorsal cavity of the spinal cord, where it connects to the phrenic nerve -a branch of the cervical plexus- and then goes on to innervate several organs, such as the heart and lungs.

Since the vagus nerve travels throughout the body and helps regulate heartbeat and breathing, it is considered a vital part of the autonomic nervous system. The vagus nerve consists of two main components: the vagus cranial nerve and the spinal vagus nerve.

The vagus cranial nerve -also known as the tenth cranial nerve- is the longest of all cranial nerves. It extends all the way from the brain stem down to the neck and regulates the heart, gastrointestinal tract, smooth muscles, liver, gallbladder, and spleen.

The vagus nerve has two main branches, the left, and right vagus nerves. The left vagus nerve passes through the neck, where it joins with the phrenic branch of the spinal cord (via a ganglion). The phrenic branch then descends to join with the diaphragm muscle.

The right vagus nerve passes through the neck and then splits into two parts, one going to each side of the heart. It then descends down the trunk, passing below the diaphragm muscle before branching into a small bundle of fibers that run down either side of each lung and connect them together at their bases.

The main job of these fibers is to control breathing. When you inhale, they send signals to increase pressure in your lungs so that more air can enter them; when you exhale, they send signals to decrease pressure so that less air escapes from under your ribcage.

FUNCTIONS OF THE VAGUS NERVE

The vagus nerve is a cranial nerve that carries sensory and motor information from the internal organs to the brain. It is responsible for parasympathetic inner-vation of most of the organs in the body, including the heart, gastrointestinal tract, respiratory system, smooth muscles, and glands -the parathyroid gland and adrenal glands.

The vagus nerve also helps regulate blood pressure via vasodilation. When you experience stress or anxiety, your heart rate increases as your sympathetic nervous system takes over to provide you with more energy. When this happens, the vagus nerve sends a signal through your bloodstream telling your digestive system to slow down so that it can stay at rest while your heart pumps faster. This reduces the amount of oxygen flowing through your veins and arteries, which can help lower blood pressure.

The vagus nerve is a cranial nerve that conducts impulses from the brain and spinal cord to the heart, gastrointestinal tract, and smooth muscles. It is involved in regulating heart rate and blood pressure, digestion, and coughing. It has several functions, but here are the main three:

1. Providing sensory input to the brain - This function allows your body to receive information from its environment and send it back to your brain.

2. Providing motor output to your heart and lungs - Your heart and lungs use this information to determine how much oxygen they need and how hard they should contract in order for you to survive.

3. Controlling certain bodily functions - For example, you may use this pathway when you sneeze or cough in response to something that disturbs your nasal passages or respiratory tract (for example).

Here is a list of some of the other many functions of the vagus nerve:

- The vagus nerve relays signals from the brain to other parts of the body.
- The vagus nerve regulates heart rate and blood pressure by affecting the heart and lungs and, therefore, how fast one's heart beats and how much blood flows to different parts of the body.
- The vagus nerve helps regulate digestive processes by controlling food digestion, secretion of digestive juices, and contraction of smooth muscle cells in the intestines.
- The vagus nerve helps to regulate breathing patterns and has a role in digestion.
- The vagus controls heart rate, blood pressure, and other functions of the body by sending signals from the brain to the heart through nerves in your neck that travel along with the vagus nerve.
- The vagus cranial nerve helps control digestive processes such as vomiting and stomach acid production through sensory input from your gut.
- The cranial nerve vagus carries sensory information from the face, eyes, nose, throat, and ears to the brain.
- The spinal nerve vagus carries motor information from the lungs and heart to muscles throughout the body.
- The vagus nerve carries signals throughout the body. The signals are sent from the brain to various organs throughout the body via sensory nerves.
- The vagus nerve is responsible for controlling heart rate and digestion. It also plays a role in regulating the central nervous system, intestinal function, and blood pressure.
- The vagus nerve senses touch, temperature, vibration, pain, pressure, and chemicals in your body through receptors located on its surface. This allows you to feel when something is touching or pressing against you or when something is hot or cold against you.
- The vagus nerve controls sweating by affecting the glands that make sweat.
- The vagus nerve can also affect other organs indirectly through its connections with them.
- The vagus nerve helps control blood pressure by regulating the flow of blood through arteries and veins.
- The vagus nerve helps control breathing by controlling the rate at which air passes through the lungs during inhalation and exhalation.

- The vagus nerve also helps regulate blood glucose levels by sending signals from pancreatic beta cells to insulin-producing cells in your pancreas.
- The vagus nerve communicates with the stomach to help us feel full when we eat.
- The vagus nerve also plays an important role in our immune system. When we're sick or injured, it sends messages to the white blood cells that cause them to come out of their resting place -the spleen- and travel throughout our body, fighting whatever infection or injury we've gotten ourselves into
- Providing somatic information to the heart
- Providing parasympathetic stimulation to the heart
- Providing somatic information to the GI tract
- Providing somatic information to the smooth muscles of bronchioles and larynx -the voice box

VAGUS NERVE DYSFUNCTION

The vagus nerve is a bundle of nerve fibers that runs from the brain to the heart and lungs. It works like a sort of "brake" on your heart, slowing it down when you need to rest or slow down your breathing.

A vagus nerve dysfunction is a disorder that disrupts the normal function of the vagus nerve. The vagus nerve is a major nerve in the body, carrying information between different parts of the brain and organs, as well as between different parts of the body. It is also responsible for controlling heart rate and blood pressure, helping to regulate digestion and breathing. When things go wrong with your vagus nerve, you may experience symptoms like excessive sweating, muscle twitching, trouble swallowing or speaking, dizziness and fainting, and even heart palpitations.

The vagus nerve is made up of two main branches: one that connects to both lungs; another that connects to all internal organs except the stomach and large intestine -which are connected via another pair of nerves. When something goes wrong with either one of these branches, it can have an impact on other systems in your body; for example, if there's an issue with your lungs' ability to breathe properly, then you won't be able to get enough oxygen into your blood system which can cause dizziness; if there's an issue with digestive acid production then it will not be able to break down food properly which could lead to nausea or vomiting; if there's an issue with heart rate.

When this nerve is damaged or dysfunctional, you may experience symptoms such as dizziness, chest pain, and trouble swallowing. The vagus nerve also has connections with your digestive system, so when it doesn't work properly, it can cause nausea and diarrhea.

Vagal nerve dysfunction can be caused by many different things, including injury to the nerve itself or damage from an infection -like Lyme disease. You may even experience no symptoms at all if your vagus nerve is healthy!

If you think that you have vagal nerve dysfunction, talk with your doctor about testing for Lyme disease so they can determine whether or not there's an underlying cause for this problem.

CAUSES OF VAGUS NERVE DYSFUNCTION

Vagus nerve dysfunction is a condition that occurs when the vagus nerve becomes damaged. The vagus nerve is responsible for sending sensory information from the brain to the rest of the body, as well as regulating the respiratory rate and heart rate.

The vagus nerve is located in the neck, and it runs from the brain through the heart, lungs, and other organs. When there is vagus nerve dysfunction, it can cause problems with those organs. For example, if there's damage to this nerve, it can cause a person's heart rate to slow down so much that they might feel like they're stopping breathing. This can be very dangerous, and it can even lead to death!

There are several causes of vagus nerve disorder:

- Brain tumors: Tumors can grow on nerves in your head or neck and cause damage that leads to a vagus nerve disorder
- Heart disease: Heart disease can cause scar tissue to form around your heart valves which can cut off blood flow through your heart and thus cause vagus nerve disorder
- Lyme disease: Lyme disease causes inflammation in your central nervous system, which can lead to a vagus nerve disorder

If you have vagus nerve dysfunction, it can cause a number of problems for you and your health. For example, if you are sensitive to stress or nervousness, then you may experience palpitations -a fast and irregular heartbeat- due to your nervous system being overactive. This can lead to panic attacks or even heart failure. In addition, if you have been diagnosed with diabetes or hypertension (high blood pressure), these conditions may be worsened by vagus nerve dysfunction because they affect how well your heart works overall.

FOODS TO EAT TO IMPROVE VAGUS NERVE FUNCTION

The vagus nerve is a major nerve of the digestive system and nervous systems. It is also an important part of the body's immune system. The vagus nerve controls digestion, heart rate, brain function, and body temperature and can be damaged by a variety of conditions, including stroke, heart attack, cancer, and multiple sclerosis.

Now that you've learned a lot about vagus nerve function and how to improve it, it's time to look at what foods you can eat to support your body's vagus nerve health.

The first thing you should know is that the vagus nerve is a river of information flowing throughout your body. The vagus nerve carries messages from your brain, spinal cord, and other organs to every part of your body. This means that when you eat foods or take supplements that support the vagus nerve, they can help improve health throughout your body. Here, we will discuss some of the best foods for improving vagus nerve function and some tips for incorporating them into your diet.

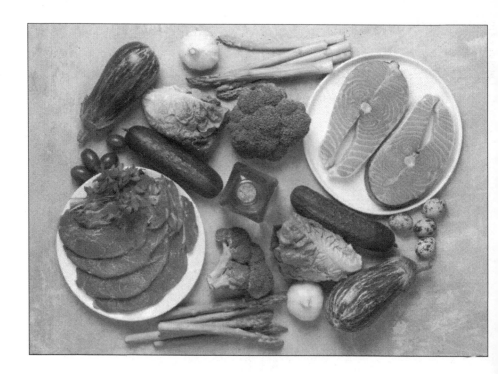

THE VAGUS NERVE plays an important role in digestion because it helps move food through your digestive system. If you want to increase the efficiency of this process, you need to eat foods that promote proper vagus nerve function. When you're suffering from a condition that causes nerve damage, it can be difficult to know what foods you should eat to improve your vagus nerve function. Luckily, there are a few easy steps you can take to make sure that your diet is as healthy and well-balanced as possible.

The first thing you should do is pay attention to what kind of foods you're eating. If you eat too much salt or sugar, for example, your nerves are going to suffer. So try not to eat too much sodium and avoid sugary snacks like candy and soda.

In addition to paying attention to what kinds of foods you're eating, also make sure that they're high in nutrients like proteins, vitamins, and minerals. This will help strengthen the nerves so they can continue working at their best level possible!

The **vagus nerve** is a long, twining nerve that connects your brain to your organs. It's an important part of the nervous system, and it can be damaged or even severed, which can cause a number of problems. Fortunately, eating certain foods can help improve the function of your vagus nerve, including:

- Oatmeal
- Berries
- Bananas
- Black beans
- Whole grains, especially brown rice
- Eggs
- Nuts (especially almonds)
- Lean meats, including chicken and turkey
- Fish

Eating foods that are rich in vitamin B6, such as bananas and avocados, can help to improve vagus nerve function and reduce anxiety.

Here is a break down of foods that are known to help improve this nerve's function and what exactly they do:

- **Cucumbers**: Some studies show that eating cucumbers can reduce inflammation in your body. This could help repair damage to the vagus nerve caused by conditions such as cancer or multiple sclerosis.
- **Garlic**: Research has shown that garlic has anti-inflammatory properties and may also help repair damage to the vagus nerve caused by conditions such as cancer or multiple sclerosis.
- **Bamboo shoots**: Bamboo shoots are another good source of antioxidants that could help reduce inflammation in your body, which could help repair damage to the vagus nerve caused by conditions such as cancer or multiple sclerosis.
- **Blueberries**: Blueberries have proven to be a great source of antioxidants, which can help reduce inflammation in your body. They also contain anthocyanins, which have been shown to lower blood pressure and help lower cholesterol levels.
- **Sweet potatoes**: Sweet potatoes have a high concentration of beta-carotene, which is a type of vitamin A that has been shown to reduce inflammation in the body and improve heart function. It also helps prevent cancer and age-related macular degeneration (AMD).
- **Eggs**: Eggs have a high concentration of choline, which is an essential nutrient involved with memory formation and learning ability. Choline also supports brain development and nerve cell health; it's especially important for children who may be developing early signs of autism or ADHD.
- **Ginger root**: Ginger root contains gingerols -compounds that have anti-inflammatory properties- as well as shogaols and zingerone, which have antioxidant effects similar to those of vitamin C or E.

OTHER WAYS TO IMPROVE VAGAL FUNCTION

As mentioned earlier, the vagus nerve is one of the main nerves in the body that connects the brain to the heart. It's also known as the tenth cranial nerve, and it has two branches, the right and left vagus nerves. The right vagus nerve is responsible for controlling the heart rate, and the left vagus nerve controls your digestive system.

Since both of these functions are vital for your overall health, it's important to keep them working properly so you can stay in good health. Fortunately, there are several ways to do so:

- Exercise regularly

- Eat a healthy diet
- Get enough sleep
- Take supplements to boost your immune system
- Try acupuncture
- Regularly consume omega-3 fatty acid supplements, such as flaxseed oil or fish oil
- Drink plenty of water to flush out toxins from the body
- Exercise regularly, especially if you have high blood pressure or diabetes and are overweight or obese
- Make your diet rich in fruits, such as grapes, bananas, oranges, vegetables, such as carrots, broccoli, lettuce, whole grains, and lean proteins like chicken or fish instead of processed foods that are high in sodium and fats, which can damage the vagus nerve and make it less effective at sending signals to the brain that help control heart rate, breathing rate, and other bodily functions.

5

CONNECTION BETWEEN THE VAGUS NERVE AND HUMAN EMOTIONS

*A*lthough the main function of your vagus nerve is to regulate breathing, heart rate, and digestion, by doing so, it also plays an important role in regulating your emotions. You may be familiar with this process if you have ever had a panic attack or felt like you were choking on something when you were eating or drinking. This is because your vagus nerve plays a key role in controlling these functions so that you can avoid having an episode of anxiety or panic disorder.

The vagus nerve is affected by emotions in many ways. It releases hormones that affect how you feel, how you think, and how you act. When you're stressed or anxious, for example, your vagus nerve releases chemicals that increase heart rate and blood pressure. This can make it harder for your heart to pump enough blood to all of your organs, thus leading to symptoms such as chest pain, dizziness, and shortness of breath.

The vagus nerve also controls your emotions by regulating your breathing, heart rate, and appetite. It's believed that when this nerve is damaged or blocked, it can cause emotional disturbances such as anxiety and depression.

In addition to being responsible for controlling emotions, the vagus nerve also helps control how fast you breathe. When you get upset or excited, your breathing speeds up or slows down accordingly -which affects how quickly oxygen reaches your brain. The faster or slower you breathe, the more emotional changes you experience from those emotional states.

A person's emotions are largely controlled by the vagus nerve, and since this nerve connects to all the organs and glands, including the heart, lungs, gastrointestinal tract, liver, and pancreas, it carries impulses from brain stem areas to other parts of the brain and body to control a person's emotional responses.

The vagus nerve communicates with other nerves that control breathing and digestion. It also sends signals to other nerves involved in regulating body temperature and pain sensation. When these nerves are damaged or dysfunctional, they can lead to abnormal emotional responses such as panic attacks or seizure disorders.

The vagus nerve is responsive to both positive and negative stimuli from the environment around us. The signals received by this nerve help us determine what kind of responses we should have toward a particular stimulus or situation.

Also, the vagus nerve is involved in the regulation of emotions by acting on certain brain areas that are responsible for emotional learning. When afferent signals travel along this pathway, they stimulate neurons in areas associated with emotions. These neurons then influence activity in other parts of the brain that control complex behaviors such as social interaction.

For example, when you feel angry or afraid, your body produces stress hormones like cortisol and adrenaline. These hormones activate receptors on your adrenal glands, which respond by releasing more cortisol into your bloodstream. This causes you to feel more stressed out and anxious. In addition to affecting your heart rate and breathing rate, these hormones can also cause your muscles to tense up in preparation for action!

CONNECTION BETWEEN THE AUTONOMIC STATE AND DEFENSIVE BEHAVIORS

As we have discussed in chapter two above, most vertebrates have two main defense systems that kick into place whenever they feel threatened or face an attack, which are immobilization and fight or flight. These responses both require access to many body resources for them to be properly activated by the sympathetic nervous system.

Immobilization is the oldest of the response system and is possessed by virtually all vertebrates. When compared with the mobilization response, which requires a great deal of energy and resources, immobilization works well to reduce the body's metabolic demands.

Also, when compared with the fight or flight response which requires speedy activation of the sympathetic nervous system, immobilization simply requires a total shutting down of all autonomic functions in the body, and this is only achieved through a vagal pathway in the parasympathetic system.

Before the establishment of the polyvagal theory, attention was not exactly paid to the immobilization behavior, and it was assumed that flight or flight response was the only response to threat of any kind. The difficulty experienced in understanding the defense behavior was no doubt partly due to the absence of cardioinhibitory vagal tone in vertebrates and mammals whenever faced with threats. As a result, a low vagal tone was taken to be an indication of a reaction to a threat.

However, polyvagal theory sheds new light on the autonomic foundation of threat behaviors. The absence of a vagal tone. Accordingly, ventral vagal tone withdrawal in response to threat increased vulnerability to a severe dorsal vagal induced syncope that would support immobilization and remove the competition for effective sympathetic activation to increase cardiac output to support mobilization.

6

HOW TO CONTROL YOUR EMOTIONS
USING THE VAGUS NERVE

*T*o control your emotions using the vagus nerve, you need to be able to identify and acknowledge them. This is hard for some people because they don't want to admit that they are feeling a certain way. The truth is that we all have emotions, and we all feel them from time to time.

The next step is to identify what type of emotion it is. For example, when someone says, "I'm mad at you," this means that they are angry at you. If someone says, "I'm sad," then they are sad or upset about something or someone in their life.

Once you know what type of emotion it is, then you can take action on it. You might want to talk to your friend or family member about how they are feeling or why they are feeling that way. This will help them understand what has caused their anger so they can learn how to deal with their emotions in a healthy way moving forward.

However, if you keep experiencing one particular emotion over and over again, for example, depression, anger, or frustration, it may be a sign that something is wrong and needs fixing. The good news is that activating your vagus nerve can help you work on your emotions - understand and sort them out.

The vagus nerve helps modulate emotional responses by activating specific areas of the brain related to emotion regulation, such as the amygdala and anterior cingulate cortex (ACC). These regions are involved in regulating fear and anxiety responses. When activated, these areas can help you feel more relaxed or calm if you're feeling stressed out or angry. In fact, studies have shown that people who have their vagus nerve stimulated via deep brain stimulation (DBS) have improved moods with fewer symptoms of depression than those who do not have DBS treatment for epilepsy surgery.

BENEFITS OF VAGUS NERVE ACTIVATION

Apart from the emotional benefits, here are a few more reasons you might want to consider activating or stimulating your vagus nerve:

Improved Mood and Better Suited to Deal With Stress

The vagus nerve is a key regulator of the stress response. While it's not unusual to experience stress at some point in life, this can be a trigger for depression and anxiety disorders if left unchecked. By activating your vagus nerve through Vagus Nerve Exercises, you'll be able to regulate your mood and cope with daily hassles more effectively.

To activate your vagus nerve:

- Sit in a comfortable position, shut your eyes and take in a deep breath through your nose.
- Imagine that you're breathing into your belly. As you breathe out, allow yourself to exhale any tension or stress that may be lingering in your body.
- Repeat this exercise for a few minutes.
- Afterward, sit quietly and focus on your body. Feel the weight of your arms and legs against the surface that you're sitting on.

RELIEF FROM DEPRESSION AND ANXIETY

Vagus nerve exercises have been shown to help relieve depression and anxiety. People with vagus nerve disorders tend to experience more mood swings and irritability, which can make it quite difficult for them to cope with daily stress, such as commuting to work or handling a bunch of kids. Vagus nerve stimulation has been shown in research studies to decrease symptoms of depression and anxiety while improving the ability of patients to deal with their lives outside of the hospital setting.

Vagus nerve stimulation helps reduce pain by increasing activity within the brain's pain control center (the nucleus accumbens). The vagus nerve also acts as a regulator for breathing rate, heart rate, and blood pressure levels; therefore, when combined with other treatments such as medication therapy or surgery, this system may be activated, resulting in positive changes in physical health over time.

The vagus nerve stimulates the release of acetylcholine, which is a neurotransmitter that helps regulate brain function. This is why many people with depression, anxiety, and other mental health disorders have been found to benefit from stimulating their vagus nerve.

Vagus nerve stimulation has been shown in research studies to decrease symptoms of depression and anxiety while improving the ability of patients to deal with their lives outside of the hospital setting.

SLOWER RATE OF COGNITIVE DECLINE

The vagus nerve is a large nerve that runs from the base of your brain to your abdomen. It's also known as the tenth cranial nerve, as it consists of many branches that innervate multiple organs, including your heart and lungs.

The vagus nerve plays an important role in regulating our breathing rate and body temperature—it helps us breathe more deeply when we're working out or exercising vigorously, for example—but it also has connections to other parts of our body that impact cognitive function directly:

- It sends messages back down through this same pathway (called "autonomic" control) when you have a heart attack or stroke; if these signals aren't sent fast enough by this route, then they might not reach other parts of the brain where they need help protecting against injury or damage from something like elevated blood pressure levels.*
- Stimulating one side of this pathway can help improve memory functions such as remembering where you left things because all those signals are being sent at once instead of just going one way only, which means less confusion about what's happening around us."

REGENERATION OF DAMAGED ORGANS AND TISSUES

The vagus nerve is a major player in the immune system. It helps to regulate your overall health by promoting the growth of new cells and aiding in wound healing. By strengthening this part of your body, you can also help prevent certain diseases from developing over time.

In addition to helping with organ regeneration, exercise has been shown to increase levels of T-cells, which are crucial for fighting off infections or other diseases caused by viruses and bacteria. The more active you are on this front (and certainly if you're working out at home), then the better off you'll be!

TREATMENT OF EPILEPSY

The FDA approved VNS as an alternative therapy for epilepsy in 1997. Aside from epilepsy, VNS is also employed in the treatment of conditions such as severe irritability in children with autism spectrum disorders, depression and anxiety in adults, fibromyalgia, and chronic pain.

THE VAGUS NERVE CAN BE A GATEWAY TO BETTER HEALTH

The vagus nerve is a main part of the parasympathetic nervous system. The vagus nerve can be activated by breathing exercises, meditation, and other relaxation techniques. It plays a salient role in our fight or flight response, helping us to respond quickly when we are under threat or have to flee from danger.

The vagus nerve also helps regulate heart rate and blood pressure, helping us maintain a healthy lifestyle through regulating our bodies' functions at rest and during exercise. It is important to note that the vagus nerve is capable of sending signals from our brain, through the spinal cord, and into other areas of the body. This means that it can send signals both ways, which is why it can be stimulated by breathing techniques or spoken affirmations. The vagus nerve also connects with our immune system, so stimulating it can help us fight off illness more quickly.

WAYS TO STIMULATE THE VAGUS NERVE FOR BETTER EMOTIONAL HEALTH

Your vagus nerve is a major part of how you feel, and it plays a role in everything from digestion to heart rate. The vagus nerve is also responsible for activating your brain's parasympathetic nervous system (PSNS), which helps you calm down and relax when necessary. When this system isn't working properly, your body may be more reactive than usual, and this can cause stress or anxiety symptoms like increased heart rate, shortness of breath, and muscle tension.

Vagus nerve activation in its various forms has been shown to reduce blood pressure by up to 20 percent among people with high blood pressure who are not taking medication for it, and it may even decrease some types of pain! Vagus nerve activation also improves sleep quality because it reduces cortisol levels -a hormone associated with stress responses in the body that can affect memory consolidation during REM sleep cycles.

For many people, improving the communication between their vagus nerve and brain can help ease inflammatory diseases like rheumatoid arthritis, lupus, and irritable bowel syndrome.

If you want to improve your emotional health with exercise or meditation but don't know where to start, then check out these tips. The following activities will help stimulate your vagal tone so that you can increase your overall well-being:

GETTING MORE SLEEP

Getting more sleep is important for emotional health. It can be difficult to get enough sleep if you are staying up late or have a job that keeps you busy all through the day, but it's worth it. So, how much sleep do you need?

The amount of sleep needed by anyone depends on their age and activity level:

- For children between 0-3 years old, babies should be sleeping 11-14 hours per day (on average).
- For children between 3-12 years old (and adults), teens should be sleeping 8-10 hours per day on average.
- Adults generally need about 7 to 8 hours of sleep per night -the amount will vary depending on how physically active you are in your daily life. People who work night shifts may need even more because they spend less time in bed before going to work.

Tips for getting a good night's sleep:

- Keep your bedroom dark, cool and quiet. Your body will naturally want to sleep at night, so if you can, try to stay away from screens in the hours before bedtime.
- Set a schedule -go to bed and wake up at the same time every day.
- Try to get 7-8 hours of sleep every night.
- Avoid eating right before bed -it can make it hard to fall asleep.
- Don't drink caffeine late in the day because the effects can last for several hours after drinking it.

STIMULATING THROUGH THE EAR

The vagus nerve is the longest cranial nerve, and it connects the brain to the stomach and other organs. It also acts as a pathway for sensory information from the ear canal all the way down to your heart.

According to Dr. David Perlmutter, author of "Brain Maker," many people can feel a tingling sensation when they stimulate their vagus nerve through their ears with an ear device. This is because this area of your brain controls your digestive system, so when you stimulate it using an ear device -like one he recommends, you're actually stimulating yourself, not just something external like an app or video game!

You can do this by rubbing gently over either side of your neck near where it meets at the base of each ear; then gently rolling around on each spot until you feel some sort of sensation that feels like pins and needles or maybe even just warmth in those areas where there was no feeling before, depending on how sensitive you are.

BREATHING DEEPLY AND SLOWLY

Deep breathing exercises are a great way to stimulate the vagus nerve, which will help you feel more relaxed and calm. If you're new to deep breathing, start by inhaling for five seconds and exhaling for five seconds. Once you become comfortable with this level of focus, try taking longer breaths, such as inhaling for fifteen seconds and exhaling thirty-five.

This type of practice can take some time before feeling any results, but it's worth sticking with! The benefits of deep breathing exercises include:

- Decreased stress levels
- Increased oxygen intake
- Increased blood flow to the brain
- Better sleep quality
- Improved focus and attention
- Increased feelings of happiness & contentment
- More energy
- Better immune system function
- Improved metabolism and digestive health

AN ACT OF KINDNESS TO SOMEONE

As you can see, there are many ways to stimulate the vagus nerve. One of the most effective ways is by doing something kind or compassionate for someone else. This might sound strange at first, but it's true! Kindness and compassion are good for your health because they help you feel calm, relaxed, and happy. They also make you a better person who will be more likely to keep living in this world we call Earth with all its beauty and challenges.

So why should we be kind? Well, besides being good karma -and helping others out-, kindness can also be considered a form of meditation! When you're feeling down or frustrated with life situations like getting stuck behind an SUV in traffic on your way home from work every day during rush hour traffic. Or even just having bad days where nothing seems right anymore, try giving yourself a few minutes each day where no one else needs anything from anyone else except themselves, no matter what happened yesterday or today.

Just sit still with yourself until whatever comes up falls away naturally over time without needing any outside help at all. It is a great way to practice being kind and compassionate with yourself first before doing anything else. After all, if you can't take care of yourself, then how can you take care of others?

GARGLING OR SINGING OUT LOUD

If you are looking for a swift and easy way to stimulate your vagus nerve, gargling water is a great option. You can practice this by filling a glass with warm water, placing it into your mouth, and then letting it sit there for 30 seconds or so before spitting it out.

The warm temperature of the water will help relax your throat muscles as well as make them less resistant to swallowing -which means they'll be easier to clear. You may also add a slice of lemon or lime, which will help to calm your throat, clear out any mucus and improve digestion.

Singing out loud is another great way to improve emotional health, especially if you're singing along with someone else! Singing in groups has been shown to boost our happiness levels even more than when we sing alone; this may be because we feel more social while singing together -and thus happier- but also because other people around us tend not only to cheer us up but also provide encouragement during difficult times throughout our lives.

Sing out loud! If you're feeling creative, try singing a song that relates to an emotion. When I get sad or angry, I'll often listen to my favorite music playlist while I'm cooking dinner or doing household chores so that when the mood strikes me again, I'll have good music ready at hand too!

VAGUS NERVE STIMULATION (VNS)

Vagus nerve stimulation (VNS) is an implanted device that sends electrical impulses to the brain through a wire that goes directly into your chest. The impulses help to regulate your heart rate and blood pressure by speeding up or slowing down your heartbeat; they also regulate digestion by stimulating certain parts of your stomach; they slow down or speed up your breathing by interrupting the signals from your lungs to tell your diaphragm to breathe, and they can even impact emotions by modulating activity in certain parts of the brain responsible for mood regulation.

The U.S. Food and Drug Administration has approved VNS for treating epilepsy in adults and children who are more than three years old. Vagus nerve stimulation (VNS) is a treatment for epilepsy, anxiety, depression, and more. It is also used to treat pain conditions such as migraine headaches. The procedure involves placing an electrode on the vagus nerve and stimulating it with electrical impulses.

YOGA THERAPY

Yoga poses can stimulate the vagus nerve by engaging different muscle groups while stretching them open so that you feel more comfortable with your body. The benefits of yoga are many:

- It helps you relieve stress and increase flexibility.
- It improves your immune system by increasing circulation in the body.
- It provides a means to reduce anxiety by improving breathing techniques.
- And most importantly -and what I think makes yoga so powerful- it helps you build trust with yourself.

Here are a few Yoga poses that could prove useful:
Child's Pose

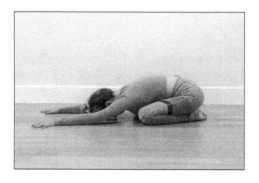

Image Source: theyogacollective.com

144

Exercise your mind and body by taking a few deep breaths while relaxing into Child's Pose.

Relaxing the body is one of the best ways to reduce stress, calm your mind and help you feel more energized. When we practice yoga postures, we tend to focus on the stretch or pain in our body, but when we take some time out for meditation, it helps us realize that all our bodies are connected, so even if there is discomfort in one area it shouldn't stop us from moving forward with our practice.

The vagus nerve connects our brain with other organs throughout the nervous system, including muscles, organs, and glands, making it an important part of health maintenance for both mental and physical well-being! This can be achieved through exercises like this which use slow controlled breathing patterns combined with relaxation techniques such as deep abdominal breathing (pranayama).

ADHO MUKHA SVANASANA - DOWNWARD FACING DOG

This pose is a great way to stimulate the vagus nerve, which plays a role in digestion and metabolism. It also stretches out your hamstrings and calves, which can help with lower back pain or fatigue. If you're new to yoga or have had any injury to your lower back, this pose will be especially helpful for you because it helps open up the chest area that would otherwise be pushed into one position by other poses like Plank Pose (aka Boat Pose).

To do this pose:

- Stand tall with feet hip distance apart, knees slightly bent at 90 degrees.
- Reach hands forward as if trying to touch down along the floor on either side of your body
- Turn palms upward -towards the ceiling
- Place both feet flat on the floor facing each other
- Engage core muscles while aligning the spine straight but not rigidly so as not to cause strain on joints
- Let the abdominals rise up between the rib cage without straining neck muscles!
- Squeeze inner thighs together tightly enough, so they don't sag downward away from the torso base line but don't lock them together completely either.

UTTANASANA - STANDING FORWARD BEND

Start with the feet hip-width apart, hands at the heart center. Inhale as you raise your arms overhead and exhale as you fold forward from the hips and lower torso to a squatting position on all fours. If this is too difficult or if it hurts to stretch out through your shoulders, place both hands on the floor behind you for support.

PRASARITA PADOTTANASANA - WIDE-LEGGED STANDING FORWARD BEND

The first thing to do is breathe deeply into your belly. Once you've taken a big breath, push the hips forward to stretch the back of your legs. Lift up and look forward as much as possible while keeping your spine straight (don't arch). Hold for 30 seconds, then release back down onto all fours again before moving on to pose 2 below!

CONCLUSION

To conclude, let us have a quick recap of all that has been discussed above. First, the vagus nerve runs from the brainstem down into your abdomen. It connects with many different organs and tissues throughout your body, including your heart and lungs. The vagus nerve also plays an important role in regulating how you feel emotionally, or do you think it's the other way around? Researchers have found that improving communication between your brain and this nerve can help ease inflammatory diseases like rheumatoid arthritis, lupus and irritable bowel syndrome. In fact, for many people dealing with depression or migraines who have trouble managing these issues on their own may benefit from improving their vagal tone first!

Next, everything you feel, from joy to anger, is regulated by your vagus nerve.

The vagus nerve is the most important nerve in your body. It's a bundle of nerves that connects your brain and spinal cord to every organ in your body, including your heart, lungs and digestive system.

The vagus nerve controls how you feel emotionally by sending messages to different areas of the brain so they can regulate emotions like happiness or sadness. In fact, it was once called "the parasympathetic nervous system" because it helps us maintain restful sleep after a stressful day at work instead of waking up feeling stressed out all over again!

Next, your vagus nerve helps you communicate with others. It's a cranial nerve that connects the brain to the heart, lungs, and other organs in your body. The vagus nerve is responsible for regulating your heart rate and breathing. When you're upset or struggling with something difficult, it can make it hard for you to talk about what's going on inside of yourself, but having someone listen can be helpful!

Furthermore, the vagus nerve is responsible for both heart rate and digestion, but the way it works can be confusing.

The vagus nerve helps regulate your heart rate, but not by affecting the electrical signals in your heart itself -that's what meds like beta blockers do. Instead, it affects how quickly your digestive system moves food through your body so that you don't get hungry or too full before you've had enough to eat.

This might seem like a minor difference—but when we talk about emotions and health conditions like anxiety and depression, often times people will say things like "I'm just anxious" instead of "I'm experiencing anxiety symptoms." This is because our brains are hardwired to process feelings first before we even think about how our bodies feel!

So, in conclusion, vagus nerve health is important for your emotional and physical well-being. It's the connection between your brain and your body that helps regulate how you feel emotionally (from anger to joy) and physically (from breathing to digestion). The next time you experience an emotion like anger or fear, think about whether it stems from something going on in your vagus nerve system, and if so, what can be done to make sure that connection stays healthy.

BONUS CHAPTERS

THE GUT-BRAIN CONNECTION & HEALING YOUR CHILD'S VAGUS NERVE

7

THE GUT-BRAIN CONNECTION

*T*he gut-brain connection, or the brain-gut connection; whichever form of the term you are familiar with, one thing is certain - this connection exists and is stronger than you probably realize. Research has shown that the brain affects gut health, and in the same way, the gut may affect brain health. Why? This is because -believe it or not- the gastrointestinal tract is quite sensitive to emotions, meaning that feelings such as anger, sadness, and happiness can trigger certain reactions in the gut. The communication between the brain and the gut is called the gut-brain connection, which is made possible through the gut-brain axis.

This explains why seeing a gory sight can immediately cause a person to throw up the content of their bellies. You've most likely experienced the feeling of butterflies in your stomach before. It's an involuntary response to stress or excitement, and it happens when your gut tells you something is right. You may have also noticed that when you're anxious or worried, your heart starts beating faster and you feel flushed in certain areas of your body -the stomach included. These sensations are caused by nerves in the gut sending signals to other body parts -like the brain- about what's happening within our bodies at any given time.

The second brain is responsible for 80% of serotonin production, which helps maintain good moods; 90% of dopamine production, which causes feelings of excitement; as well as helping regulate hunger levels through hormones like leptin -which controls appetite.

While we're all aware of the gut-brain connection, it's important to understand how that relationship works in your body. The gut and the brain are joined by nerve cells called neurons. These neurons release chemicals called neurotransmitters that travel through your bloodstream to other parts of your body, including your heart and lungs. This exchange of information between these two organs allows you to feel emotions like happiness or sadness, think logically or creatively (like solving puzzles), remember what happened yesterday -or even dream about something in the future!

The bacteria living inside our intestines can affect how we think and feel by changing levels of serotonin or dopamine in our brains, and those same neurotransmitters play a role in regulating moods as well as physical responses like hunger pangs when eating foods containing gluten -a protein found mostly in wheat products. In fact, some people report feeling less happy after eating certain foods because they disrupt this delicate balance between good bacteria vs. bad ones within their gastrointestinal tract.

The gut is a mysterious organ that we know very little about, yet it profoundly influences our mental health. Did you know that the neurons in your brain are more than those in any other part of your body? And did you know that these neurons communicate with each other through chemical signals -neurotransmitters- produced by cells called neurons? This means that what happens in your head can affect what goes on down there! So let's talk about how this works:

THE GUT

The gut is an organ that runs from the mouth to the anus. It's responsible for digestion, absorption of nutrients and water into your body, as well as regulating moods and emotions. It's also where many diseases originate, like cancer.

The gut has two major parts: the small intestine, which absorbs food, and the large intestine, where waste is stored until it can be passed out of your body through defecation or urination. The gut is lined with layers of cells that help it to function properly. These cells are constantly replaced by new ones that grow from stem cells in the intestine. But when these stem cells become damaged, they can no longer produce healthy new cells. This can lead to intestinal damage and disease.

Your gut is mostly bacterial. Your digestive system is home to trillions of microbes, which are essential for your health because they assist with the breaking down of food and produce vitamins and enzymes that allow you to digest food efficiently.

These bacteria also regulate the immune system by encouraging it to fight off harmful bacteria or viruses before they can take hold in your body. Research shows that having healthy gut flora helps prevent allergies and asthma attacks by improving immune function in children who have been exposed to certain foods during infancy. In other words, if you want your child's immune system strong enough to protect them from infections like colds or flu each year -and potentially save their life- increasing gut flora might just be worth considering!

Gut bacteria also influence neurotransmitters like serotonin and dopamine, which are involved with mood disorders like depression and anxiety. Inflammation plays a role too: studies show that people who suffer from chronic conditions such as IBS tend to have higher levels of inflammation than those without them -and this could be because inflammation increases our perception of pain by sending signals through different parts of our body besides just feeling physical discomfort alone.

HOW IS THE GUT CONNECTED TO THE BRAIN?

We know that your brain and gut are connected, but what exactly does that mean? Could it be true that your mental state is affected by the bacteria in your gut? The answer is yes. In fact, there may be a connection between how healthy our digestive systems are and how happy or sad we feel — at least according to some scientists who study this phenomenon.

You've probably heard that your gut is connected to your brain. But did you know that the microbes living in your intestines can have a strong impact on how you feel and think?

The microbiome (the bacteria in our bodies) is linked to mental health, and researchers believe it may be the key to understanding why some people are more prone to depression than others. Studies show that people suffering from anxiety or stress are more likely to have higher numbers of certain types of gut bacteria than those who don't experience these conditions. For example, one study found that women with irritable bowel syndrome (IBS) had higher levels of inflammatory compounds in their blood when compared with healthy controls—signs suggesting they were experiencing greater stress levels due to their IBS symptoms.

The gut and brain are connected in many ways. The gut has a direct influence on your mood, behavior, and sleep. It may even affect your memory or learning ability. And when something goes wrong in one area of your body, it can have an impact on another system like the brain or skin. For example, if you feel a sore throat or upset stomach that lingers for more than two weeks—it could be because there was an issue with the bacteria in your digestive tract that triggered inflammation elsewhere within your body (like perhaps at the site where food enters)

It might explain why you're dizzy when you feel sad

Dizziness is a common symptom of anxiety, depression, and PTSD. In fact, it's one of the most common symptoms people experience when they're sick or feeling down.

The reason for this is that your brain sends signals to your stomach (the gut) to help with digestion. When you feel anxious or depressed, your body releases stress hormones into the bloodstream—and these hormones can cause nausea and vomiting if they reach their target organ: your gut!

This connection between brain and gut has been shown in multiple studies over recent years — including one published last month by researchers at Northwestern University's Feinberg School of Medicine, who found that being told about negative events increased levels of serotonin in mice brains via connections between neurons known as synapses.

Where Does The Vagus Nerve Come In?

The gut-brain connection is bidirectional. Both the gut and brain have a lot to say about each other, and they can influence one another in many ways. The vagus nerve plays a main role in this relationship: it's responsible for carrying messages between your brain and your gut. This means that when you feel stressed or anxious, your vagus nerve sends signals that travel up into your cortex -the outer layer of the brain- which then triggers certain thoughts or behaviors from there, including food cravings!

As we've seen above, the enteric nervous system (ENS) is an important part of this connection. The ENS consists of neurons that connect your intestines directly with your brain and spinal cord.

The gut bacteria mentioned above produce neurotransmitters that act on the brain. These neurotransmitters are called neuroactive peptides or neuropeptides because they have effects similar to those produced by hormones such as serotonin or dopamine -they affect mood and behavior by altering how you perceive yourself or others around you.

The gut microbiota also releases hormones that affect processes such as digestion and immunity. It's also possible that these hormones play a role in mood regulation.

HOW TO IMPROVE GUT-BRAIN CONNECTION

Diet

Our diet can affect the gut microbiome. In fact, it's estimated that 50% of your immune system is located in your gut. This means that if you have a poor diet or eat foods with a lot of sugar and processed foods, you might be compromising your body's ability to fight off illness.

The relationship between your gut bacteria and how well they work together is called dysbiosis -a medical term meaning an imbalance between beneficial microorganisms (probiotics) and harmful ones (pathogens). When this happens over time, the result can be chronic inflammation, which contributes to obesity, heart disease, and other health conditions like asthma or depression.

There are many reasons why people may want to improve their diets through nutritional supplements:

- They may not get enough protein in their diets.
- They may experience digestive issues related to age.
- They need more calcium than what's available from food sources alone.

Here are a few feeding tips:

Following a moderate-fat diet.

- Eating more fat is a great way to improve the gut-brain connection.
- Fatty foods are important for brain health, as they help with the absorption of vitamins and minerals. Fat also helps with the absorption of omega-3 fatty acids, which can help reduce inflammation in your brain. Furthermore, having more fat in your diet will increase prebiotics -foods that help promote gut health. Prebiotics are found in plants like onions and garlic.

Eating fermented foods.

- Fermented foods are great for your gut. They're loaded with probiotics and prebiotics, which help feed the good bacteria in your gut and keep it healthy.
- Fermented foods can be eaten raw or cooked—if you want to try them raw, try making kimchi at home!
- You can find fermented foods at most grocery stores these days. Some examples are kimchi (Korean cabbage), sauerkraut (German), and miso paste (Japanese).

Probiotics and Antibiotics

There are many theories about how probiotics affect the brain, but one of the more interesting ones is that they can improve memory. In a small study published in Nutrition Reviews, researchers found that participants who took probiotics showed improvements on tests measuring their mental agility compared to those who didn't take them.

Probiotics are good bacteria that help with digestion and the immune system. They're found in fermented foods like yogurt, kefir, and sauerkraut. Probiotics are good for your gut. You can also take probiotics as a supplement. Probiotic supplements may help with constipation, diarrhea, allergies, and asthma -and they might even help you sleep better!

Antibiotics destroy harmful gut bacteria and can kill off beneficial bacteria along with them -which means they may not be good for everyone's mental health either. But there's hope! In fact, research has shown that restoring some of these lost microorganisms after taking antibiotics could help boost mood and reduce anxiety levels in people with autism spectrum disorder or anxiety disorders.

Reducing Stress

Stress is a major cause of GI problems. It can cause the gut to produce more mucus, which can lead to inflammation; it can also lead to changes in the gut microbiome and make you more susceptible to other conditions like irritable bowel syndrome (IBS).

To reduce stress, try these tips:

• Breathe deeply. Deep breathing helps with digestion by reducing anxiety, improving relaxation, and reducing inflammation. Try taking five deep breaths daily while lying down or sitting quietly at home, even if you're not feeling stressed! This simple exercise has been shown repeatedly as an effective way for people suffering from anxiety disorders like post-traumatic stress disorder (PTSD) or panic attacks.

Avoiding NSAIDs That Can Harm the Stomach Lining.

If you're prone to stomach ulcers and want to avoid them, it's important to avoid NSAIDs. These include aspirin, ibuprofen, and naproxen. NSAID use can cause bleeding in the stomach lining, which can lead to an ulcer or even perforation. This type of pain is often difficult for people with RA who don't have much time for rest because they may need their treatment at the doctor's office or hospital emergency room at any given moment during the day.

If you take these medications regularly, then it's important not only to avoid them altogether but also to speak with your doctor about switching over from one type of NSAID drugs, like ibuprofen or naproxen sodium, down to another type, such as aspirin instead. This is because these drugs can cause stomach ulcers that weaken connective tissue inside our intestines, causing symptoms of the leaky gut syndrome, including bloating, diarrhea, constipation, heartburn/acid reflux, etc.

Getting Enough Sleep.

Getting enough sleep is important for a healthy gut. Sleep deprivation can cause digestive problems, including constipation and diarrhea. If you're not getting enough sleep, it's time to start making adjustments in your life.

• Set up a routine for going to bed and waking up at the same time every day -like 7 p.m- so that you don't have trouble falling asleep or staying asleep throughout the night if something comes up during your normal bedtime hours or early morning wake up times.

• Try using an alarm clock that isn't so loud so that it won't disturb your sleeping patterns as much as traditional clocks do.

• Avoid using caffeine late in the afternoon/evening before sleeping; try drinking some tea instead.

- Try eating foods high in magnesium like nuts, seeds, avocados -which contain 18% RDA of this mineral per serving- and bananas.

Conclusion

In summary, there are many ways to improve the gut-brain connection without medication. The first step is to get to know your gut and how it works. If you are worried about your gut health, don't hesitate to consult with a doctor or nutritionist who can help you get on track with the right lifestyle changes for your unique body type!

8

———————————————————

HEALING YOUR CHILD'S VAGUS NERVE

HEALING YOUR CHILD'S VAGUS NERVE

our child's vagus nerve is a critical part of their health. If it isn't working properly, your child might experience some of the following symptoms:

- Irritability and anger
- Depression and sadness
- Anxiety and nervousness
- Low self-esteem or lack of confidence
- Headaches and migraines

Now, all parents want the best for their children, but this goes beyond sending them to the right schools and giving them everything they want. It includes the ability to sense when most of their emotional and physical responses are as a result of a dysfunctional vagus nerve and how to heal and activate this vagus nerve to give them better health statuses.

The vagus nerve is a long nerve that goes from your brainstem to the heart and lungs. It's responsible for controlling your heart rate and regulating breathing. When you're healthy, this process works well -but if you have a weak or damaged vagus nerve, it may not work as well as it should.

158

When we talk about strengthening a child's vagus nerve, we're referring to what happens when the child is trying to relax. For instance, when a child takes deep breaths to slow down their heart rate -heart rate variability. This is beneficial because whenever there's an emotional response in our bodies like stress or anxiety, there's also some kind of physical response like increased blood pressure or body temperature, and these responses can cause further damage by stimulating our muscles even more strongly through reflexes like breathing faster than usual!

To heal your child's vagus nerve, help your child achieve the following physical exercises:

STEP 1: BREATHING

Breathing is a great way to calm down and relax. When you breathe, your body and mind are able to release stress. You can teach your child to do this by taking deep breaths through their nose while counting to 4 or 5, then exhaling slowly through pursed lips and counting to 4 or 5.

If your child finds it difficult to count to 4 or 5, you can let them start with a smaller count of 2 and slowly work their way up.

As they are breathing deeply, teach them to focus on releasing tension from every part of their body, including those places that aren't usually associated with tension:

- Behind the eyes or jaws
- Under the arms
- In between shoulder blades
- At the base of the neck -the base chakra
- Under each shoulder blade
- Along each side rib cage -or wherever else it may be.

This particular act of releasing tension may not be easy, but with time and constant practice, your child should get the hang of it in no time and begin to see results. Remember, it is important to practice breathing exercises with your child to ensure that they feel supported and do them correctly.

STEP 2: PRACTICING COMPASSION AND SELF-CARE

In the second step of this process, you and your child will practice compassion and self-care.

Compassion is a skill that can be learned. Aside from being a virtue you'd want your kids to have, it could also positively affect their health. You can start this by teaching your kid to take care of themselves by eating well, getting enough sleep, and exercising regularly. Remember, true compassion always starts with oneself.

Self-care is important because it helps reduce stress which can lead to increased seizures in some people who suffer from epilepsy or any other condition. There are many ways we can take care of ourselves without needing medication:

- Meditating
- Doing yoga
- Reading books on mindfulness
- Exercising regularly
- Spending time outdoors

You may also want to consider joining a support group for parents with children who have epilepsy or other chronic health conditions if yours is suffering from one. This will give you an opportunity to talk with others who understand what it's like as a parent of someone with these diagnoses, and hopefully make some new friends too!

Because children naturally have short attention spans, it is your responsibility as a parent to try and find ways to make these activities fun for your kids.

STEP 3: LAUGH

Laughter is good for the heart, soul, and mind. It's also a quick way to release endorphins that help a person cope with pain or stress.

The vagus nerve is responsible for sending signals from the brain to the muscles so they can respond appropriately when something occurs in the body. When you laugh, it stimulates this nerve and sends signals down through the body into the heart, where they cause an increase in blood flow there, allowing more oxygen to reach tissues like those around the lungs and heart muscle itself. This increased amount of oxygen helps us feel better! Laughing also releases dopamine which helps us feel happy and less stressed out by allowing us to relax.

To heal your child's vagus nerve, engage them in activities that are sure to make them laugh. This could be anything, ranging from a day out on the beach, picking flowers in the garden, or watching their favorite cartoons.

STEP 4: HUM

Humming is a great way to relax and calm down. It's easy to do anywhere, at home or in the car, so you and your child can take advantage of the situation wherever it presents itself. You can hum quietly or loudly, it doesn't matter! Just make sure that your voice isn't raised when humming so as not to disturb others around you.

Humming helps people feel calmer because it stimulates the vagus nerve, which helps control heart rate and blood pressure levels by slowing down its contractions throughout our bodies; this means we can slow down our breathing patterns without even realizing what we're doing until later on when we start getting more relaxed naturally due in part because of how well this technique works!

So, if your child is experiencing a bad day, all you have to do is sit them down, and together, you can hum the tune of your favorite songs.

STEP 5: SING

Singing is a great way to improve mood, which is especially important for children who have vagus nerve issues. It can also help you relax, sleep and focus. Singing can reduce stress by releasing endorphins in your brain that make you feel good about yourself.

Singing is one of the best and most enjoyable ways to relieve stress and can be even more effective when you do it with others. If you have children at home, try singing with them or taking them to a musical event.

Conclusion

The vagus nerve is a critical part of your child's nervous system. It helps regulate heart rate, digestion, and other body functions. The vagus nerve can be damaged by stress or trauma. The good news? You can strengthen it through relaxation and breathing exercises! We hope these tips prove helpful for you and your child.

Made in the USA
Monee, IL
27 June 2024

60823006R00104